# HIDDEN CAUSES
## of HEART ATTACK
## and STROKE

*Inflammation, Cardiology's New Frontier*

## by Christian Wilde

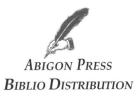

**ABIGON PRESS**
**BIBLIO DISTRIBUTION**

ISBN: 0-9724959-0-8
SAN: 254-8542

**Publisher's Cataloging-in-Publication**
*(Provided by Quality Books, Inc.)*

Wilde, Christian.
    Hidden causes of heart attack and stroke :
    inflammation, cardiology's new frontier / by Christian
    Wilde. — 1st ed.
        p. cm.
    Includes bibliographical references and index.
    ISBN 0-9724959-0-8

    1. Coronary heart disease—Etiology—Popular works.
    2. Myocardial infarction—Etiology—Popular works.
    3. Cerebrovascular disease—Etiology—Popular works.
    I. Title.

RC685.C6W544 2003                     616.1'23071
                         QBI03-200146

PRINTED IN THE UNITED STATES OF AMERICA

Fifth Printing February 2007
5 7 9 10 8 6

Cover Design: Knockout Books
Book Design: Rosamond Grupp
Edits and Index: Peter Stokes, Ph.D., USC
Illustrations: Young Park

"Much of what Christian Wilde suggests today, is destined to become standard medical practice in the next decade. No other reference—so succinctly discusses the myriad of ways we can prevent the heart attack or stroke that is always lurking over our shoulder."

—*Gregory Guldner, MD., MS., F.A.C.E.P*
*Director, Emergency Medicine Residency Program*
*Loma Linda University Medical Center*

"I have just finished reading your extensive chapter on fibrinogen. You have been visionary in your early identification of what may well turn out to be, **the next major breakthrough** in stroke and heart attack prevention. After my more than 50 years in the medical profession, you have even opened my eyes. I am convinced that the information you present will save many lives."

—*Ronald Lawrence M.D., PhD.,*
*appointed advisory member of four*
*Government National Boards, including*
*the Institutes of Health and founder of*
*the American Medical Athletic Association*
*Author of* **The Miracle of MSM**

# COMMENTARY

*John A. Rumberger, Ph.D, M.D., FACC*

There is an expression from the first known book on medicine that I show at the beginning of all of my lectures. This is an exact copy of the ancient Chinese and its translation.

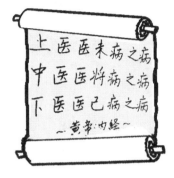

It was written by Huang Dee, long before Aristotle or Hippocrates and by some one whom we, in Western or European literature, have never heard of; and yet it crystallizes the concept of Preventive Medicine.

---

Superior doctors prevent the disease.
Mediocre doctors treat the disease
    before evident.
Inferior doctors treat the full-blown disease.
--Huang Dee: Nai-Ching
    (2600 BC First Chinese Medical Text)

---

When a patient goes to their doctor, the purpose normally is to learn the origin of their symptoms or complaints, and to get advice about medication or a cure for the problem. The patient seeks education from the doctor although the doctor may personally be ignorant of the particular medical condition itself or any contributing issues. When it comes to discussing prevention, since the disease is NOT evident, it is often put on the "back burner" while other more immediate health issues require consideration.

For heart and vascular disease prevention, the patient is told to watch their cholesterol, get some exercise, and eat a healthy diet. These are so called "population" goals and although worthy advice for all of us, they are often stated in a matter of fact way with no details as to how these might be applied or altered for a given individual. Often these recommendations are not strongly emphasized to the patient, little true information or education is imparted and like the doctor, the patient often puts any action on this advice as well "on the back burner."

The issue then, for the patient, is to take charge of his or her own destiny. The best way to do this is to be educated in plain and simple language about prevention and the factors that contribute to heart and vascular disease development. Until *The Hidden Causes of Heart Attack and Stroke*, a reliable resource for the patient was simply not available, as the subject is vast and complicated.

The good news is that 80 to 90% of heart and vascular disease risk can be accounted for by a variety of inherited metabolic and lipoprotein [that is "cholesterol"] disorders. However these disorders are contributed to or abrogated in a given individual by environmental, lifestyle, dietary, and exercise choices and are probably also mitigated as well by a variety of common and uncommon infectious diseases. These risks can be refined through routine and advanced lipoprotein and metabolic blood testing and by simple, direct, and safe plaque imaging, such as what is accomplished with Electron Beam Tomography. The question is for most: *"How can I learn about these things and know what may be best for me?"*

Although I have not actually met Christian Wilde, I know him very well. We have communicated often over the past four plus years, beginning during my tenure as a

*Professor of Medicine* at the **Mayo Clinic.** The information that he presents in this tome is a reflection of his personal journey of education. Christian, faced with a problem that he did not know, did not even expect that he had, has devoted himself to research to learn the cause or causes of his own situation. In educating himself about heart and vascular plaque, he has provided the benefit of allowing *you to also be educated.* The style of his writing is comfortable and conversational and yet the information that he delivers is vitally important and up-to-date.

Christian now shares his expanding knowledge with all of us and there are lessons here that would be of benefit not only to patients but *clinicians* as well. The thirst for knowledge continues and all of us need to be students. Perhaps, in this developing world of education for prevention, to paraphrase Huang Dee, the *"Superior Patient Helps Prevent the Disease Before Evident."* The best way to prevent disease is to educate the patient and provide him or her with an empowerment to accomplish this goal in conjunction with his or her own doctors. Christian Wilde indeed is helping us all take the first step in becoming "Superior Patients."

Respectfully Submitted,

*John A. Rumberger, MD*

John A. Rumberger, Ph.D, M.D., FACC
Former Clinical Professor, Mayo Clinic
Clinical Professor, Ohio State University

## DISCLAIMER

Nothing you will be presented in this book is designed to replace or supercede your doctor's advice or treatment plan for you. The information is meant to be a reference source and an educational tool. If you have been diagnosed with heart disease or have previously experienced a heart attack or stroke and if you would like to minimize additional risk, your doctor may find the information from highly respected researchers and physicians helpful in reducing further risk. Medical information is updated continually and what one may read that is represented and accepted today may be challenged in the near future. All any author or researcher can reasonably do is to present the information from reliable sources as it appears in the literature. It is not the intent of the publisher to provide all of the information available on any given subject; you are encouraged to seek additional information. The purpose of this book is to aid you in a better understanding of the diagnostic and treatment options that may be available to you as the patient and to prepare you for discussions with your physician. The publisher and author shall have neither liability or assumed responsibility for any adverse reactions, alleged or actual damage caused by any information provided in this book in regard to any entity or individual.

# TABLE of CONTENTS

# FOREWORD

There is simply nothing more devastating than the sudden, unexpected loss of a loved one. For too many Americans, this loss comes at the hand of heart disease. Cardiovascular disease (diseases of the heart and blood vessels) accounts for more than 50% of all deaths in this country. Each year 1.1 million Americans have a heart attack. 370,000 will die of this attack… 250,000 of them will die within one hour of suffering their heart attack.

Decades of research have taught us that much of heart disease is preventable. We know that the major risk factors for heart disease are advanced age, smoking, high blood cholesterol, high blood pressure, diabetes, and family history. Certainly we can do nothing to change our age or our family history, but we can, and have done a great deal to reduce the incidence of smoking, to reduce cholesterol levels and to treat high blood pressure and diabetes in this country. We have also learned that being overweight and being sedentary predispose us to heart disease, so we have counseled Americans to maintain an optimal body weight and engage in regular physical activity. Because of the information gained from this research, and the public health efforts we have instituted to educate Americans about heart disease, we have been able to decrease the incidence of heart attack and stroke in this country over the past several decades. Unfortunately, despite the gains that have been made, we are still in the midst of an epidemic of heart disease. Despite our best efforts, more clearly needs to be done. As a practicing cardiologist, I have seen many people suffering heart attacks despite having optimal blood pressure and cholesterol levels, having normal body weight and exercising regularly. These individuals do not smoke, do not have diabetes, and have no family history of heart disease. So what goes wrong? Well more recent research has indicated that there may be a number of risk factors for heart disease that we are only now just discovering. These risk factors include additional cholesterol particles that standard cholesterol tests do not measure, inflammation and inflammatory proteins and other proteins and chemicals in the body that have been known for some time but whose connection to heart disease hasn't been elucidated until recently. As a researcher and cardiologist I fully understand that the more we discover about heart disease, the more we have yet to learn. Many of these new "emerging" risk factors for heart disease are well known in cardiology and research circles, but many patients, family members and even some physicians do not yet have access to this information.

*Fortunately, there is now a book* that clearly and concisely explains these new and emerging risk factors for heart disease, which can help patients and family members as well as the public more fully understand a little more about heart disease. Most of us have a personal story or have been touched by heart disease at some point in our lives. For many of us the results have been tragic and heartbreaking. As research in this area advances, public information needs to keep up. This book will inform many people about the most current, cutting edge research about heart disease.

Karol Watson, M.D., Ph.D
Co-Director of Program in Preventive Cardiology
Director of Lipid and Hypertension Management, UCLA

# INTRODUCTION

The *Hidden Causes of Heart Attack and Stroke* was not only written to help you minimize your risk of heart disease and stroke but also to benefit individuals who have already experienced prior events. The information you will read will help you in becoming a more proactive, empowered patient; able to present your case intelligently when interfacing with your doctor. You will very shortly become intimately familiar with diagnostic blood tests that <u>for the first time in medical history</u> are able to guide your doctor, in identifying many of the inherited mechanisms. Hidden inherited mechanisms that even now may be silently threatening your life and eventually your children's, as co-inheritors of genetic heart attack and stroke risk factors. The good news is that once these mechanisms are identified, the only remedy is often found in natural medicine. If, however, you assume you can take a passive back seat role by simply believing the doctor is aware of all the latest breakthrough information, you may be disappointed. Much of what you will be presented will not be routinely applied in doctors' offices for several years. The research community is 15-20 years ahead of the practicing office and what you will learn, will now put *you* on the "cutting edge." It might surprise you to know that eighty percent of the dysfunctions you will learn about are not identified with routine blood work ordered during your annual physicals. Can you or I—or our families—afford to wait? You are the guardian of those you love. Should you not become a knowledgeable advocate in your own family's healthcare?

*The Hidden Causes of Heart Attack and Stroke* will be your guide. You may not as yet be aware of it, but heart disease or stroke will ultimately affect every one of us. If not directly, then indirectly, through our parents, grandparents, spouses, our own children or dear friends. Unfortunately, one out of every two deaths in our country will be attributed to some related form of heart disease—and no one is immune.

Experience may have taught us a great deal about our particular business or our favorite hobby. We know exactly what constitutes good instruction and good business practice. However, when it comes to the most important aspect of our lives, our health, most patients are inhibited and intimidated because of a lack of knowledge, causing us to refrain from asking even the basic questions. Reticent of appearing stupid, we just nod our collective heads indicating, "whatever you say doc." Sound familiar? We are struck with "white coat fever."

It is my sincerest hope that after absorbing the information you will be presented in this book, **gathered from many of the most applauded and respected physicians, scientists and researchers,** you will become very aware of your own cardiovascular system, having learned much of the relevant medical terminology and thereby feeling far less intimidated. You will be prepared to ask well-informed, intelligent questions about diagnosis and prevention. While cholesterol is vitally important, it is not all, *just* about cholesterol, and as important as what the book will teach you about inflammation, it is not all *just* about inflammation. There are many other contributing factors which you will read about in *Hidden Causes of Heart Attack and*

*Stroke*. Any one of them in your particular profile could be the *Achilles heel*, therefore you need to be aware of the full spectrum of risk factors. The information is not meant to alarm you; the only thing that should be alarming is walking around with an undiagnosed, untreated time bomb in your body. We are taking on the number one killer in our nation, and no holds are barred. You have a huge stake in this fight. Why, in this day of advanced technology and science, should something as miniscule and seemingly insignificant as a tiny clot of blood be allowed to destroy an entire family's happiness? Why in this day of modern medicine should this intruder be allowed to steal a father, grandparent or mother away from her children without even so much as a warning? **How dare this enemy be allowed to invade your life or mine!** The *Hidden Causes of Heart Attack and Stroke* will lead you on this preventive journey.

# Chapter 1

# Who's *Winning the Battle for Your Arteries?*

If you believe your cholesterol is all you need to worry about—think again. Were you aware that 50% of all the people who experience heart attacks have had so called "normal" cholesterol?

Did you know that 80% of heart disease disorders go *undetected* by the routine blood tests physicians customarily prescribe for their patients? Statistics like these, which (in part) come from the American Heart Association, make it abundantly clear that something else besides cholesterol may indeed be ravaging one's arteries. *"The Hidden Causes of Heart Attack and Stroke"* explores not only important lipid cholesterol information, but brings to the reader much of the latest information on *inflammation* and inherited factors and how these might be equally significant causes of heart disease, stroke and premature death.

With the occurrence of 1.1 million heart attacks a year in America—and more than one third of the victims not surviving—no contributing source or diagnostic test should be overlooked. **Every 33 seconds, some one will suffer a heart attack and fifty percent of these victims will not have had warning prior to the attack.** Most certainly, as we will see, *cholesterol is not the only area of concern.*

> **80% of heart disease patients have the same blood cholesterol values as those <u>who do not</u> develop heart disease.**

**This book will address in depth other "hidden" factors that lie undetected within this 80% parameter.** How often have you heard of or even known an individual who, in spite of receiving an exemplary passing grade on their yearly physical, still became stricken or actually died as the result of a heart attack? Their physical may have even included a nuclear treadmill stress test. I can immediately recall several such instances. **One example is a young golfer who folded like an umbrella** during a routine round on the links with his friends. His golfing partners were later to explain that their buddy had told them he had passed a perfect physical evaluation just the week before. Five days later: gone! The doctor's exact words following his physical exam (according to one friend) had been, "I only wish I was in half as excellent shape as you." Be careful what you wish for!

**A 32 year old Southern California man** who had been given a clean bill of health following <u>his</u> annual checkup the previous week, was found dead in his car from a massive heart attack. The autopsy attributed this unfortunate circumstance to a *plaque rupture* (plaque hemorrhage) which had resulted from a progressing accumulation of cholesterol deposits.

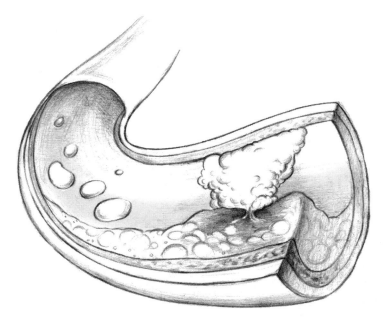

**Fig 1: Plaque rupture and clot formation**

This individual's situation had been even further complicated by undiscovered elevated *fibrinogen* (a blood clotting factor) that intensifies clot formation. It had literally sealed this patient's fate. **A lady in her mid-fifties** was not considered a good candidate for a treadmill evaluation because her cholesterol was only slightly over 200. This same lady in her prime subsequently suffered a heart attack and died two days later. The cause? Occlusion (blockage) of the left main artery. It would later be learned (by autopsy) that she actually had two other significantly narrowed arteries and an unrealized inherited LP (a) trait that by itself had **increased her risk of heart attack by more than 4 times.** Not one but two different doctors had told this patient that her problem was *stress* related. Adding to this patient's risk profile had been a highly elevated C-reactive (CRP) level for inflammation (a recently recognized marker we will discuss in great detail that can significantly increase one's risk of heart attack and stroke). If this patient had been given a nuclear treadmill, would it have alerted the doctor of the impending threat in time for intervention? Would a preventive physician have included a 10 or 16 dollar CRP test on this patient's annual physical and detected the ongoing inflammatory condition in time for antibiotic treatment? Might she be alive today and enjoying her time with her children if only these three tests had been done? Probably. The case histories go on and on and any doctor speaking candidly could add to the list similar examples that he or she has encountered in their own practice or been privy to in their medical community. *You will learn about these lifesaving tests just mentioned and several others throughout this book.* In still another dramatic example, a doctor had just congratulated his 56-year-old patient on his successful physical. This same man never made it home. He was struck down, collapsing and ultimately dying in his wife's arms as the two were walking down the steps leaving the clinic. Why? **What warning sign went undetected? Were there unidentified <u>multiple factors</u> that in combination may have triggered these events**? What you will read will hopefully lessen the chances of this happening to you or someone close to you. Physicians are often just as perplexed as the family members by such events. These health practitioners are in the business of saving lives, and such occurrences are devastating to those doctors who dedicate their own lives to helping others. Certain medical professionals will admit that they discuss such cases between themselves privately over lunch or coffee breaks. "What happened? My patient showed no indication of what was about to occur." These concerned doctors, unable to explain their patient's cardiovascular events, shook their collective heads and wondered what was missing in their diagnostics that could have prevented these catastrophies. Perhaps the patient had exhibited warning signs that were overlooked. **Most probably the new tests that we are about to address were never performed.** What may be most alarming is the possibility that the doctor wasn't even aware of their significance or their availability. It has recently been widely established and accepted that heart disease, more often than not, is attributable to a *combination* of factors that escape detection during most well intentioned physician examinations. *Do you know if you or your family members are at risk from these undetected risk factors? Have you been tested? Is your doctor familiar with them?* Will your healthcare provider pay for the newer tests? **Are you in fact, aware of these *silent* inherited heart attack risks?** It would be prudent to learn which diagnostic tools are available and why this potentially lifesaving information is worth knowing. The old adage *"what you don't know won't hurt you"* would not apply here. Early proper diagnoses, using all the diagnostic tools now available, could save innumerable lives, sparing families needless emotional agony and expense. Early, complete "leading edge" diagnoses would certainly reduce the number of required hospital stays, angioplasties and open-heart surgeries. The physician who wants to approach healthcare from the preventive standpoint will focus on obtaining and maintaining proper cholesterol levels, and exploring the inflammatory and inherited risks long before surgical intervention becomes a necessary course of action. The time for PREVENTIVE CARDIOLOGY in its true sense has arrived.

*Immediately the question arises: "But isn't all this just exactly what physicians are doing?"* Well, a growing number are, and these doctors are to be commended, but by and large too many don't even want to hear of the things you are about to learn. Here is one possible explanation why many senior doctors resist change.

*"IMPORTANT SCIENTIFIC INNOVATION RARELY MAKES ITS WAY TO GRADUALLY WINNING OVER ITS OPPONENTS. WHAT DOES HAPPEN IS THAT ITS OPPONENTS GRADUALLY DIE OUT AND THE GROWING GENERATION IS FAMILIAR WITH THE NEW IDEA FROM THEIR BEGINNING"* —Max Planck

As one doctor explained it, "When I have to add those things to what I already have on my plate, I will. In the meantime I have enough to worry about." This kind of thinking could take 15 years to change. Meanwhile patients and their families could be exposed to unnecessary anguish. At worst, there is the real possibility of needlessly shortening a productive life. Notwithstanding the fact that the emphasis has been on reducing high levels of cholesterol, there is new information (which we will explore) that suggests very low *total* cholesterol may also be problematic and dangerous. Sometimes it looks like the patient just can't win. In actuality, what you don't know and, perhaps more importantly, what your doctor hasn't discovered about your particular *total risk profile* could prematurely shorten your life. If you think this is an overly dramatic assessment, consider how many friends and acquaintances are missing from the high school or college reunion rolls because of heart disease. With each gathering, heart disease continues to be the leading cause of the diminishing numbers. While many doctors still tolerate a cholesterol level of 245 or 255 as not being a serious cause for concern...

***The average person admitted to a hospital with a heart attack statistically has a total cholesterol of 220.***

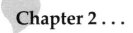

Chapter 2 . . .

# Who's Minding the Store?

## FAILURE OF PHYSICIANS TO REACH THEIR OWN STANDARDS

A study published in the June 1998 issue of the *Archives of Internal Medicine* determined that **"most patients with cardiovascular disease in primary care** (under close supervision) were not receiving cholesterol screening and management as recommended by the *National Cholesterol Education Program* guidelines." The institution labeled the circumstance, **"A failure of physicians to reach their own standards."** The study had discovered:

1. One-third of the patients had not been referred to cholesterol screening.
2. Forty-five percent had not received any type of dietary counseling.
3. Over two-thirds (67%) had not been prescribed anti-cholesterol medication.

The study included 603 heart patients and involved 159 doctors. *Most importantly, only 84 patients (14%) with cardiovascular disease had achieved the recommended LDL (the "bad" cholesterol) level of less than 100 mg/dl.* Patients innocently but ignorantly believe they are following and are receiving proper advice when heart disease patients with LDL levels of 125/ 135 and possibly higher are being accepted as normal levels. An LDL level of 100 would be a safer level than what has been generally accepted as normal for heart disease patients. Setting even a target goal of 85 (according to many of the leading proponents such as Dr. Robert Superko), would be advisable if one seriously wanted to *regress* the effects of years of buildup in the patient's arteries. Doctors are anxious to suggest this level for their patients *after* the heart attack, why not before? People in parts of China, where heart disease and cancer are extremely rare, have an average LDL in this very range (under 85) and total cholesterol of 160-140 or lower. Why would a lower level not be something for all patients to shoot for? Among all the physicians surveyed, cardiologists were reported to take the most conscientious care in checking a patient's cholesterol levels and monitoring their blood pressure. Cardiologists are also reportedly more active in discussing lifestyle changes that might lower their patient's risk of heart disease. Again, the cardiologists received high marks for prescribing blood pressure medication as well as cholesterol-lowering drugs to patients who would benefit from them. In comparison (according to a Boston MA study), **"primary care physicians as a group, do not appear to have the same standards."** Boston doctors Randall S. Stafford and David Blumenthal found, in reviewing the records of some 30,000 office visits involving 1,521 US physicians, that doctors only monitored their patients' blood pressure 50% of the time. Isn't blood pressure called the "silent killer" because there is no warning? What was also significant was that these **doctors measured their** patients' **cholesterol levels only 4.6% of the time!** Advice on stopping smoking was offered in 3% of visits, weight loss in just 5.8%, and exercise according to Stafford and Blumenthal, was only discussed in 11.5% of the office visits. In a press statement, Dr. Stafford offered the following conclusion, reported in the 11-98 edition of the *Journal of the American College of Cardiology*:

> *Even among cardiologists, the overall level of services provided, tended to be quite low* **and other physicians fall even shorter of the goal. I think we need to enhance the training or continuing medical education of primary care physicians."**

*If after 30-40 years of undeniable evidence as to the importance of controlling cholesterol is not being respected among the very professionals who are entrusted with our healthcare... what would lead us to believe that the newer lifesaving methodologies and diagnostics will be applied today in doctors' offices?*

If you have an open-minded, leading-edge physician in your corner, consider yourself a lucky individual—but *how would patients know whether they are getting leading edge advice?* Hopefully, what you will be presented will answer that question. The evidence has shown there are too few physicians breaking the new ground. Most resist additions to their already demanding practices, and still the incredible information continues to astound even the most astute practitioners. *Fifty percent of all heart attacks occur in people with normal cholesterol readings.* We should all be able to agree that something is obviously being missed.

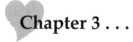 Chapter 3 . . .

# *Heredity*

## YOU HAVE INHERITED HEART DISEASE!

Based on the knowledge available 10-20 years ago, it was ominous news to hear the doctor say, "You have inherited heart disease!" The end-point, the final result, would have seemed inevitable. The profession knew <u>some-thing</u> had been inherited, but in a great number of cases they were at a loss to identify the actual *individual* factor or factors that were dysfunctional. The end result was of course recognized as heart disease. In contrast, today, with all the knowledge and advanced diagnostic testing capabilities that a physician has at their beck and call (if they will use them), heart disease discovered early, need not be as dire as it once was. With all the new clinical trial evidence emerging, and with all the supporting science, it is a vast oversimplification to use only the catch-all term, "inherited." *The most practical and obvious question that has begged to be asked all along is...*

# WHAT SPECIFICALLY HAS BEEN INHERITED?

There, it has finally been asked. In retrospect, if the physician of the past had the benefit of today's newest information, he or she could have possibly surmised that **THE PATIENT HAD INHERITED ONE OR MORE RISK FACTORS OR "MECHANISMS",** *and if these individual mechanisms were not identified and controlled, their presence would result in the development of heart disease.* Having said that, it is not contradictory to acknowledge that heart disease is, more often than not, attributable to a genetic, *inherited condition.* It is also true that one or more of these *inherited genetic conditions,* not neutralized, would eventually be responsible for a great percentage of heart disease development in individuals *regardless of their cholesterol readings.* As a matter of fact, Dr. Superko, in the publication *Preventive Cardiology* in 1998, made reference to a Genest, Martin-Munley study which appeared in *Circulation* in 1992; which *had found genetically linked dyslipidemia (lipid dysfunction) in 77% of 101 CAD patients.* In further confirmation of the genetic link, the report also identified an inherited dysfunction found in 54% of the patient's first and second-degree relatives. We will see that among the 50% of people who present with normal cholesterol and still have heart attacks, much of their risk will be defined somewhere within this genetic parameter.

## BUT IT MUST HAVE BEEN INHERITED

How many times has a doctor, unaware of the actual cause of a patient's fatal heart attack, explained to an inquiring family member that their loved one's death had been caused by something inherited? That single word, *heredity*, has always sounded so final and so indefensible. That explains it! **That one word, absent any further explanation, was expected to suffice. Heredity!** Thank you doctor, if it was inherited, there was probably little that could have been done to avoid it! While it is accurate to say much of heart disease is genetically inherited, it is possible today, with the new diagnostics, to actually identify many of the *individual inherited mechanisms* before they produce the first heart attack or stroke. To explain it away as "heredity" after the fact, after the heart attack, is counterproductive and part of a process that is fundamentally flawed. To doctors like M.D., Ph.D, Karol Watson, Co-Director for *Program in Preventative Cardiology and her staff* at *UCLA* and other preventive leaders in the field, the benefits of the new approach are obvious and vital.

> Unfortunately, many of the recently discovered causes for heart disease are still overlooked in too many physician examinations.

How many doctors, for instance, actually order a CRP blood test on a patient's physical to learn if an infection is present, or test a moderately high cholesterol profile for LDL and HDL sub-fractions, or look to an LP (a) test to identify an inherited dysfunction? How about your physician? Of 12 physicians interviewed only one was even aware of the importance of most of these newer risk factors just *two and half years ago*. One physician commented that he believed 90% of the physicians in the country did not know of the importance of all the markers we were talking about, and he was honest enough to add, "and neither do I." That was a little over two years ago. That percentage has been changing a good deal with the publication of study results introducing diagnostic procedures and new concepts from the groundbreaking work of physician leaders like *Paul Ridker, Michael Miller, Russell Ross* (deceased), *Robert Superko, Antonio Gotto, Rene Malinow, John Rumberger, Michael Gaziano, Steven Nissen, Charles Hennekens* and *Meir Stampher to name but a few, each leading the way to newer* and better science and application in diagnosing and treating heart disease. Their work is being ever more widely acknowledged. What is different about this preventive approach is that the doctor's focus is on preemptive identification of the actual "inherited mechanism," as opposed to accepting the counter-productive, but popular, safe harbor all encompassing explanation of...*heredity.*

## "I WON'T MAKE 50"

Most patients in the past, upon hearing, "you have inherited heart disease," would have been inclined to feel they were confronting a situation totally beyond their, and their doctor's, control. Perhaps a father, uncle or other close relative had died prematurely of a heart attack and the son or daughter began looking at their own mortality and counting their days. Has anyone ever told you that they expected to die young? If you asked them how they arrived at such a negative prognosis, the answer might have been something like, "well, Uncle Joe died from a heart attack when he was 47, my dad had an early fatal heart attack and Aunt Julie had a massive stroke at 53, so I've always wondered if I would even see 50." Their thinking process would have been influenced by the accepted idea that heart disease is inherited and consequently there probably isn't too much one could do to alter the inevitable outcome. In actuality, the following could have been possible.

> **Their loved ones had needlessly, prematurely died of complications produced by a specific individual unidentified silent heart attack risk which today could have been diagnosed and treated.**

**Do you know if you carry such risk?** It is not an overstatement to say that the application of new scientific information could save your life, or that of someone you care deeply about.

## EXCERCISE AND DIET

Three or four weekly trips to the gym and a low-fat diet are definitely important steps in the right direction, but they do not give one immunity from the risk factors we are addressing. There are already hundreds of excellent books available on diet and exercise offering helpful advice. **Exercise is of vital importance, and even for those who cannot maintain a vigorous regimen, 5 or 6 thirty-minute walks a week have shown remarkable reductions in cardiovascular or stroke events and lowered blood pressure.** These benefits cannot be ignored—however, it would not be accurate to assume heart disease could be totally avoided if one simply exercised and ate right.

# AN IMPORTANT DISTINCTION:

## "HEREDITY" IS NOT USED IN THE CONTEXT WITH CONGENTIAL BIRTH DEFECTS AS IN MORE THAN 100 CARDIOVASCULAR DISORDERS

Our discussion focuses on heart disease as it pertains to lipid and inflammatory management in relationship to heart attacks and strokes. It is imperative to understand that this is our area of concentration, because while there are congenital inherited birth defects as in *hypertrophic cardiomyopathy* or any one of a myriad of other *congenital* heart diseases, *The Hidden Causes of Heart Attack and Stroke* addresses the detection of individual lipid and inflammatory "mechanisms." The important difference between the two classifications ("inherited" and "congenital") is that "congenital" may refer to a physiological defect manifested at birth or in earliest childhood development, while inherited factors take their toll progressively *over a very long period of time until they result in a diagnosis of what we know as heart disease.* Our focus will remain on the second distinction.

*What we are exploring does not negate cholesterol's role. On the contrary, it is important to understand that the presence of any of the mechanisms we are discussing is exacerbated when found in combination with complicated cholesterol markers, including elevated triglycerides.*

As we will see, deviations in proper cholesterol markers in combination with inherited and inflammatory risks only hasten and further complicate one's overall risk.

# BUT MY DOCTOR SAID MY CHOLESTEROL IS NORMAL

Hopefully it is, but even with normal cholesterol you or a loved one may still be at risk for heart attack or stroke. Perhaps you are thinking, *well, my doctor checks my cholesterol yearly, so are all these new diagnostic tests really necessary?*

It is not one or the other. **IT IS THE FULL DIAGNOSTIC PROFILE THAT HAS BEEN MISSING.** It is *cholesterol* together with *inherited and inflammatory markers* that must be evaluated and treated and brought into compliance.

Most of us, after 25 years of discussion of cholesterol numbers and ranges have become fairly familiar with cholesterol. It would be helpful to review the latest updates on cholesterol from the most respected medical leaders before exploring the inherited mechanisms and the area I have chosen to call, *inflammation—cardiology's new frontier.*

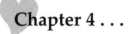

# Chapter 4

# Cholesterol
## The Good, the Bad and the Ugly

### 220 CHOLESTEROL CAUSES HEART ATTACKS

The average cholesterol level among patients admitted to the hospital suffering a heart attack was not 300, or 265, or even 240, as one might expect. No, according to a national study, the average total cholesterol score was actually 220.

### 150 AN IDEAL CHOLESTEROL LEVEL?

**William Castelli,** one of the directors of the Framingham Heart study, has said that cholesterol levels of 150 or lower almost guarantee immunity from heart attack. Of some 5,000 subjects whose history he followed for 25 years after the initial Framingham Study, **not one has had a heart attack or died of heart disease.** These statistical results speak volumes.

It is common knowledge today that a 150 total cholesterol count is considered advisable by physicians and
attainable by patients who have had a first heart attack. As
a point of common sense, then, shouldn't a lower number
than 200 be the mark to shoot for everyone? Since it is
incumbent upon patients to lower their total serum cholesterol to 150 after a heart attack, wouldn't a number
below 200—perhaps 160-180 have been a good target before the first heart attack, thereby averting the catastrophe
in the first place? Based on Castelli's findings, would a
lower overall cholesterol level be a recommendation that
would better safeguard the general population? It would
be foolish denial to take refuge in the fact that not everyone experiences heart disease.

**While it is a fact that not everyone is prone to heart
disease, how would you or I know which of us falls into
the safe or unsafe category without being properly tested
for the hidden risk factors?** How would your physician
know? There are doctors who dismiss the newer information clinging to the advice they gave 30 years ago. "All you
need to do is eat three good meals a day and exercise."
While there is some truth in the advice, it is woefully
incomplete. If you wonder where this type of thinking
comes from, consider the following 1828 comment.

*"MOST MEN ... CAN SELDOM ACCEPT THE SIM-
PLEST AND MOST OBVIOUS TRUTH IF IT OBLIGES
THEM TO ADMIT THE FALSITY OF CONCLUSIONS
WHICH THEY HAVE DELIGHTED IN EXPLAINING
AND HAVE WOVEN THREAD BY THREAD, INTO
THE FABRIC OF THEIR LIVES"* **Tolstoy**

## SUPPORTING DRUG THERAPY

There have been studies that have indicated many people with so-called "normal" cholesterol levels **would still derive benefit from taking cholesterol-lowering drugs. Dr. Antonio Gotto,** currently Dean of *Cornell Medical College,* along with his former colleagues in San Antonio Texas conducting the *Air Force/Texas Coronary Atherosclerosis Prevention Study* (AFCAPS/ TexCAPS), had established the following results.

**Mevacor reduced the risk of "first coronary events" including heart attack and stroke by 36 percent** *in subjects who appeared to record <u>normal</u> cholesterol levels.*

These statistics confirmed a specific reduction of 36% in a woman's risk, and a 34% lesser but still significant reduction of risk in men. There was also a welcomed 43% reduction of high blood pressure risk among those study participants who had initially presented with hypertension.

*///* **THE RESULTS OF THIS STUDY CARRY PROFOUND IMPLICATIONS FOR MANY ADULTS WHO THINK THEY ARE AT LOW RISK OF HEART ATTACK** *///*
—*Antonio Gotto*

*"Even if your LDL or so called "bad" cholesterol is **considered average**, you may still be at risk if your HDL, or "good" cholesterol (as we have come to know it) **is too low**."*

> This was the first time a clinical trial had shown that any drug could prevent a first heart attack in both men and women who have an average total cholesterol level, _but lower than normal high density HDL lipoprotein levels._"

The _lovastatin (Mevacor)_ study was a study involving some 6,000 patients across all ethnic groups. These findings may be something you would want to discuss with your doctor. This trial information might enable you to present your case for discussion more convincingly. Have you noticed how pharmaceutical companies are spending millions of dollars on television ads suggesting patients speak to their doctors about medications like _Zocor, Lipitor, Celebrex, Vioxx, Plavix_ and a host of others? The pharmaceutical houses have taken their fight to the public. A great deal of information is being disseminated through health newsletters, magazines and television, and you will continue to learn even more about other risk factors and corrective therapies over the next few years. As wonderful as the statins are, however, bear in mind that it is very important to monitor and report any muscle soreness or tenderness. Although rare, there are cases when individuals have developed a form of nerve damage known as neuropathy. While certain ailments can definitely contribute to neuropathy, such as diabetes, kidney disease and even thyroid dysfunction, it is the connection with statin drugs that is of concern. Report any symptoms such as numbness, tingling, a difference in sensitivity to weather conditions or muscle pain. Neuropathy is in its own right a very painful and regrettable condition. That said, the general consensus is that the benefit of statin therapy far outweighs the risk.

## TRIGLYCERIDES AND HDL

When a patient presents with an even moderately elevated triglyceride level and an associated low HDL, the doctor might choose to treat and modify the ratio between the HDL and triglycerides by administering a *fibrate* drug instead of a statin. Why? Because prescribing a statin drug, as effective as they are for elevated cholesterol, probably would not rectify sufficiently the imbalance for those patients whose triglyceride and HDL relationship was in serious discord. *The one overall statin drug approach is not the answer for all patients.*

Without raising the low HDL and or lowering elevated triglycerides the on-going progression of atherosclerosis is permitted to continue. A few years pass, the patient might experience a heart attack or stroke, become a candidate for angioplasty or open-heart surgery, and everyone wonders why. Dr. Michael Miller, Associate Professor of Cardiology at the *University of Maryland,* would be one doctor who would probably not be surprised at this outcome. In focusing on the results of his study we should be aware that *the accepted reference range most laboratories have been using for triglyceride evaluation is 200 as the low mark, and 400 as high.* Now consider the recommendations gleaned from the work and research of *Dr. Miller, Dr. Gaziano,* and their respective research teams.

## HIGH TRIGLYCERIDES,
### 300% GREATER RISK

**"High triglycerides alone increased the risk of heart attack nearly three-fold"** (as reported in the journal *Circu-*

*lation)*. Those study participants who were recorded as having the highest ratio of triglycerides to HDL cholesterol had *16 TIMES THE RISK OF EXPERIENCING A HEART ATTACK* as those with the lowest ratio. Another study whose results support the appeal for lower triglyceride levels appeared in the publication *Archives of Internal Medicine* as reported by Dr. Jorgen Jeppeson (associated with *Glostrup University*).

> This study determined that men between ages 53-74 who smoked and who *admitted to being physically inactive* still, BECAUSE OF THEIR LOW TRIGLYCERIDES AND HIGH HDL CHOLESTEROL, *DID NOT SHOW* A HIGH RISK OF HEART DISEASE.

*Fibrates, fish oil and niacin* all provide outstanding results in both lowering triglycerides and elevating HDL. Exercise, widely known, also raises HDL but this study indicates that EVEN THOSE MEN WHO *DID NOT EXERCISE,* STILL SHOWED A SIGNIFICANTLY LOW RISK FOR HEART DISEASE. One shouldn't, however, walk away from this encouraging information believing one doesn't need to exercise. There are many undeniable advantages to be gained from exercise at all ages. There is even more revolutionary information concerning HDL and triglyceride risk ratios. Consider...

*"THE RATIO OF TRIGLYCERIDES TO HDL WAS THE STRONGEST PREDICTOR OF HEART ATTACKS, EVEN MORE THAN THE LDL/HDL RATIO"*

This was reported by **Dr. Michael Gaziano**, Director of Cardiology and Epidemiology at *Harvard Medical School*. Normally in analysis of your blood and mine, attention has been primarily focused on the HDL/LDL ratio. The study findings suggest to even the most skeptical that this triglyceride/HDL relationship may be much more critical than previously believed. How long will it be before information as important as this becomes accepted by the medical community at large? Can you afford to wait?

## FUEL TO THE FIRE

According to Dr. Michael Miller **"ANY LEVEL (of triglycerides) ABOVE 100"** appeared to increase the risk. "It is not like cholesterol, where the higher the level, the higher the risk." The emphasis is on ANY LEVEL ABOVE 100. It took 40 years for the medical community to fully adopt the use of the stethoscope. It took some 29 years before high levels of homocysteine became recognized as a major contributor to heart disease. The list of examples of delay is endless. Finally, the long debated issue of what are acceptable parameters for triglycerides should be re-evaluated and efforts made to more stringently control levels, according to the findings of these respected physicians and their teams—and there are many more similar trials that support these findings. Miller went on to say, *"This study is the first to look at such an acceptable lower level of triglyceride. It turned out to be an important predictor of future heart disease."* In a letter to the *American College of Cardiology*, the doctor recommended that guidelines for desirable triglyceride levels be set lower. In 2001 (a year after this entry was added to the book), movement was made to lower the accepted reference range for triglycerides. Bravo!

Based on this information, should you be content the next time you hear the results of your blood tests, if your doctor tells you your triglycerides are "within range," or should you be asking which scale of reference is being used in the evaluation? The old scale, or the newer recommendations advocated by Dr. Miller and Dr. Gaziano? It is a pretty safe assumption that many practicing physicians have considered triglycerides to be a factor only when they increase beyond 400 - 500 or even 700. Consider the advice of Dr. Gotto, in regard to HDL cholesterol as he addressed a group of professional doctors concerning cholesterol and coronary risk under the *Cleveland Clinic Foundation*. According to the doctor,

**"THE ACCEPTED GUIDELINES CURRENTLY BEING OBSERVED BY THE MEDICAL PROFESSION IN GENERAL, ARE IN FACT, TOO LENIENT AND THE CURRENTLY ACCEPTED GUIDELINES ARE NOT CRITICAL ENOUGH."**

His address concentrated in part on the High Density (HDL) evaluations.

According to the doctor's report, the accepted 35 mg/dl for men was inadequate; the standard cut-off should be 45 mg/dl for men and 50 mg/dl for women.

Each point of increase in HDL score affords the patient a 2% reduced risk of heart attack. Therefore an attainable 10 point HDL increase would lower your risk a significant 20%. **Incidentally, because of these new recommendations, the chart range is currently being adjusted on most laboratory reference scales.** The new values regarding HDL and triglycerides would suggest that a patient who previously had an HDL of 35 would have been 10 points too low. This patient had therefore been exposed to unnecessary added risk. Particularly if the triglycerides were more than 100. Why has 35 been considered an acceptable low for HDL when 34 (a single point difference) was the number that suddenly got the doctor's attention and a call for action? Recalling Dr. Gotto's recommendations, the determinant for a man's HDL would be adjusted to 45, a full ten points higher. Drs. Miller, Gaziano and Gotto are like E.F. Hutton advisors: when they speak, people listen!

## THE HEART ATTACK TRILOGY:
## PREDICTOR
## OF TRIPLE THREAT

*" **If you have high triglycerides, high LDL and low HDL, you have what is associated with the highest degree of risk!***"*

—*Antonio Gotto*

The doctor explained, *"This is a much higher risk than just having high LDL alone."* Many people fall in this category.

## TRIGLYCERIDE "SPIKING"

A little discussed phenomenon has recently become another focal point of attention in the prediction of heart attack and stroke. Triglycerides suddenly rise as they circulate through the blood stream up to four hours following ingestion of a high fat meal (such as a festive dinner, or consumption of certain fast foods). Doctors have always known that there is an increase in incidents of cardiovascular episodes following heavy dining, particularly during the holidays.

## HOLIDAY FEASTS AND HEART ATTACKS

Coming out of the AHA annual Scientific Sessions were the results of a study which included 1,986 men and women who had experienced a prior myocardial infarction (heart attack). The study was performed at *Brigham and Women's Hospital* in Boston. The subjects were asked what their eating program had been during the 26 hour period prior to their heart attack. While 10% said they had eaten a "heavy meal" within the timeframe, another 25%—(15% more)—confirmed they had their attacks *just two hours* after consuming their heavy meal. This two-hour window correlates with other studies which have pursued the same issue. A study released in November (just in time for Thanksgiving dinner) began:

**"Indulgence in high-fat food raises the likelihood of a heart attack even after a SINGLE fatty meal."**

An individual who does not have a problem with their trigyceride levels would not have the same risk as someone already in the higher ranges. A study performed at *Royal Veterinary and Agricultural University* in Fredericksberg, Denmark appeared in the journal *A.T.V.B.* This research concluded that those individuals on a high fat diet experienced *post-dining hikes* at levels of 60% in triglycerides within the hours immediately following the meal when compared to their counterparts who had consumed a low fat meal. Someone with an already high triglyceride level of 500 cannot afford a hike of an additional 300 or more points.

## HOW TO NEUTRALIZE THE "SPIKE"

If one took 800 mgs of vitamin E and 1000 mgs of vitamin C prior to eating a large holiday, or any high fat, meal, he or she could significantly reduce the risk of triglyceride "spiking," reported a *University of Maryland* study.

## LOWERING TRIGLYCERIDES AND RAISING HDL BY NATURAL MEANS

Triglyceride levels respond *very definitely* to weight loss; with even as little reduction as 5-10 lbs. Most assuredly, exercise, particularly aerobics achieves impressive results. The advice you have no doubt heard is to consult with your doctor before entering into any strenuous workout program. Also, there are several natural supplements that have garnered significant patient benefit.

*Dietary therapy:* Omega 3, from fish or flaxseed oil, produces outstanding lowering effects on triglycerides, at the same time favorably increasing HDL levels. Flaxseed oil, has shown however, to produce somewhat inferior results to salmon oil for cardiovascular benefit. Be warned that one may gain as much as 25 lbs. over a year if one does not calculate the additional calories from daily ingestion of fish oil. Mackerel, tuna, salmon, trout and herring are five kinds of fatty fish that are high in omega 3. Canola oil, oatmeal, and legumes also produce excellent results. If your diet consists of 60% or more of carbohydrates, you may be experiencing high levels of triglycerides. It is common knowledge among practitioners that middle girth (pot bellies) and upper body weight can play a big part in triglyceride elevation. For those with high triglyceride levels (with a doctor's approval), the addition of the very effective niacin therapy brings remarkable lowering results at the same time significantly raising HDL. I have found it helpful to take an aspirin one half hour prior to ingestion of niacin—it helps diminish the "flushing" (a feeling perhaps best described as what a woman might experience with "hot flashes"). For additional relief include in the combination *Inositol,* particularly if you are taking 1,000 mgs or more of niacin. Be aware that initially even small amounts of niacin may cause some irritation with flushing. The best advice offered is to take the niacin with food and work up the higher dosage from modest beginnings of 25-50-100 mgs. *Caution:* large amounts of nicotinic acid should only be taken with your doctor's knowledge and approval. Therapeutic doses are above 1500 mgs; at higher levels niacin can become toxic. It is advised that liver enzyme levels be monitored just as with any cholesterol drug. Note that there are two different types of niacin: one is the immediate release form, and the second is the "sustained" or what is sometimes called "timed" released or "flush free." This type performs particularly well in raising HDL. As a matter of interest, before the advent of the statin drugs, niacin was the drug of choice for lowering cholesterol.

## NIACIN AND TRIGLYCERIDES/HDL RATIO THERAPY

The following information was released as the conference statement from *the National Institutes of Health Consensus Development Conference*, which was held six years ago and dealt with the issues of triglyceride, high-density lipoprotein, and coronary heart disease. The group convened to discuss appropriate levels and acceptable therapies for countering elevated lipoproteins, triglycerides and low HDL levels. **They concluded exercise could account for a 10-20% increase in HDL.** Quitting smoking would also increase HDL. Niacin (nicotinic acid) was recognized as a very beneficial aid in lowering triglycerides, as well as raising low HDL levels. The majority of members attending determined that weight control was an effective way both to lower triglycerides and at the same time to raise HDL. The conference participants concluded that there was significant correlation between both triglycerides and HDL in determining the *particle size* as well as the quantity of HDL particles that circulate through the blood. The smaller the particle size, the more destructive. (*see chapter 10*)

## HDL AND STROKE

Men with coronary heart disease may be at increased risk for stroke if their blood levels of HDL cholesterol are low according to a study concentrating on HDL, published in the October 97 issue of the journal *Stroke*. *The study claimed that the men at risk did not have elevated total cholesterol levels or high LDL.* These men also proved to have arterial blockages in the legs, indicating peripheral artery disease (PAD). **There is added risk of developing this form of heart disease among patients with low HDL.** Raising low HDL levels is of major importance as more and more studies have confirmed. Special attention must be directed at monitoring the risk of peripheral artery disease in both the carotid arteries and disease development in the legs.

## THE JAPANESE AND CHOLESTEROL

The Japanese, who averaged a total cholesterol range between 120-140, were rarely succumbing to heart disease until they adopted the Western diet. Very soon after doing so, their cardiovascular and cancer risk increased matching the risk of people in America. In parts of China, where a total serum cholesterol level also averaged the same as the Japanese, an almost ZERO rate of both coronary or diabetes disease was recorded. A very interesting study appearing in *Circulation* in 1997 may explain further why the Japanese have a lower cardiovascular death rate, even though the plasma cholesterol among the adult population has actually been increasing over the past 30 years.

The reason for the low rates, according to Dr. Dwyer, Dr. Iwane and their team was: **a relatively high HDL to total cholesterol ratio.**

## CAN CHOLESTEROL LEVELS ACTUALLY BECOME TOO LOW?

Who would have thought it? There is another emerging side to this cholesterol argument. There are recent studies whose conclusions indicate that a level of cholesterol can definitely drop dangerously low. This new trial information is dramatic in nature and would certainly seem (based on the evidence), worthy of further exploration, and deserving of public awareness. All the focus and concentration has up to now obviously been on lowering the lipids, but in contrast there are many studies whose results have warned that in fact cholesterol *too low* may be very nearly as dangerous as high cholesterol, particularly in regard to *hemorrhagic* stroke. A *University of Minnesota* study exploring and identifying certain life threatening dangers that appeared to be caused by very low cholesterol examined 350,000 healthy men. Dr. James Neaton and his associates reported the following:

"**Very low cholesterol proved to be similarly as harmful as very high cholesterol. Notably, there was shown to be a two fold increase in the number of deaths caused by bleeding and a 3 times increased incidence of liver cancer *believed* to be the result created by very low cholesterol."**

After twelve years of study **the final information also confirmed that participants with very low cholesterol were five times more likely to die of alcoholism.** *Another study has mentioned depression as a byproduct of very low cholesterol. Suicide rates and chronic obstructive lung disease deaths have also been reported significantly higher than normal.* Perhaps the numbers of suicides, deaths from alcoholism, and the many cases of depression as recorded by the studies all result from an absence of a certain amount of cholesterol that the body requires to function properly. It is a fact that the body must manufacture a determined amount of cholesterol to meet basic requirements. *Is it a possibility for future study that while cholesterol-lowering drugs are manipulating a safe threshold mechanically,* **over-prescribed doses** *of statins and/or fibrates are suppressing the body's natural ability to counteract and adjust dangerously low levels as one's body normally would?* There seems to be a magic number being tossed around by several proponents of the low cholesterol theory. It is very hard to find immediate acceptance for findings such as these when they are newly introduced, particularly when the medical profession and the public's mindset and focus has been conditioned to consider only high cholesterol. *But when several newer studies corroborate and confirm similar findings of previous studies, the information becomes even more difficult to dismiss.* Now, here is the kicker! Dr. Rodriquez, in a presentation at the AHA, cited this statistic:

---

**A 55% increased heart attack risk among those in his study whose cholesterol was below 160!**

---

By way of confirmation, a study out of San Diego previous to Dr. Rodriquez' report **also found the <u>exact</u> same threshold of 160 total cholesterol mark as a safe level.** Although this information illuminates a different side of the cholesterol picture it does seem to cast reasonable doubt and warn against being too aggressive in lowering cholesterol. Other research regarding low cholesterol levels has shown an alarming increase in death from several **other illnesses, including colon cancer.** It is not at all unreasonable to think that a patient learning they have high cholesterol and given a prescription for a cholesterol-lowering drug, might strive to lower their cholesterol even further through additional measures, including the elimination of many fatty foods, and dramatically increasing exercise levels. The combination of the administered prescribed statin drug with the added measures can result in overcompensation and a dangerously lowered final cholesterol level—a level lower than even the doctor may be aware of. Some physicians check a patient's level after 30-60 days, and may not again for the better part of a year or longer. On the other hand, if the Asian countries with a cholesterol level of 120-130 are not having these health consequences, where does the truth truly lie?

# IS LOW CHOLESTEROL CAUSING SERIOUS ILLNESS?

*Or is it the Illness that is Causing Low Cholesterol?*

A *Low Serum Cholesterol and Mortality* presentation at the *Society for Epidemiology* at the 27th annual meeting in Miami Florida in June of 94 addressed whether *low* TC caused a higher increase in catastrophic illnesses including an increased risk of death from *esophageal,* and *prostate cancer.* Interestingly, in contrast to other studies, this particular study did not attribute non-cancerous liver disease, and death from suicide and trauma, to low TC. The study conclusions were that certain serious diseases *cause total cholesterol to decrease,* and therefore in the opinion of the authors **the noted increase in disease was the CAUSE and lower cholesterol actually the subsequent EFFECT.** Obviously it remains a controversial subject worthy of more study.

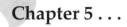

Chapter 5 . . .

# Heart Disease Begins *in a* Child's Teenage Years

Autopsies performed on young Americans have shown that atherosclerosis and the actual development of fatty streaks and plaques are found among very young subjects. The presence of this earliest form of heart disease is exactly what leads to actual heart attack or stroke as the individual matures. The heart attack in a 40, 50 or 70- year-old does not develop overnight, it took years. Call it a check that had been written 4 or 5 decades earlier only to be cashed at the much later date.

> **Dr. Steven Nissen, Co-Chair of the Cardiology Division of Cleveland, Ohio and leading authority on IVUS (intravascular ultrasound) technology determined that one in six teenagers actually has some degree of atherosclerosis in progress.**

According to studies, these abnormalities are present even among the very youngest teenagers.

You might have read about the degree of atherosclerosis detected in the arteries of young men who had died in the Viet Nam war. Many soldiers even as young as 18 had presented with very definite advancing heart disease.

> In general, autopsies of 2,976 young Americans who had died of various causes (not related to heart disease) whose ages ranged from 15-34 were shown on postmortem examination to have fatty streaks and advanced lesions already formed in the coronary arteries.

These alarming statistics were obvious even among those youngsters aged 15-19, and according to the study these lesions had "increased rapidly in prevalence and extent during the 15-34 year age span." These statistics, which appeared in JAMA, the *Journal of the American Medical Association*, advised:

> **Heart disease prevention, "must begin in early childhood or adolescence."** *Atherosclerotic lesions were found in 100% of the aortas* **(the largest artery in the human body).**

Plaques (it was reported) were also found in 50% of the right coronary arteries that actually supply the blood to the heart itself. The recommendation of the Nissen study was that the advice physicians give middle-aged patients **should also be given to the younger generation as part of a preventive educational program.** This would include stopping or (better yet) not even starting smoking, maintaining ideal weight, exercising, and eating a healthy diet.

Young people also need to become aware of their cholesterol, and monitor and control high blood pressure. A research team from the *University of Louisiana Medical Center* in New Orleans also concluded from their study that the black population was more likely to have extensive fatty streaks in the arteries, but went on to conclude that raised lesions were common in both black and white people alike. No one skates clean here. Dr. Jack P. Strong, the lead doctor in the study, gave the following advice:

*"It is going to take more than just the doctors...it's the parents, it's the schools, it's the students and the young people themselves knowing that they need to start early."*

Strong concluded by saying, "that's the main message."

## A SERIOUS RISK TO CHILDREN

To say our children are at risk for heart disease is a pretty revolutionary statement inasmuch as we as a society have only looked to heart disease as a product of middle age. The facts support this new approach, and hopefully will alert parents and serve as a wakeup call to young people. Weren't we all invincible once? Dr. Nissen, and his researchers had also evaluated plaque in the arteries of some 300 deceased subjects whose donor organs had been *harvested* from youngsters who had died by dramatic situations. The *donor hearts* were being readied for implantation as replacement hearts in patients whose hearts were in rapid decline. The doctor's findings confirmed a large degree of atheroclerotic disease in a very significant number of the young deceased subjects.

> *The report was alarming, showing that 17% of patients 20 years of age, 60% of patients between 30-39 years of age and 71% between the ages of 40-49 showed obvious coronary artery disease in progress.*

The doctor added another piece to the cardiovascular puzzle when he made the following statement:

**"Patients who die of a plaque rupture when they are 45 years old probably have had the disease since they were teenagers."**

## STATIN THERAPY FOR YOUNGSTERS WITH (HeFH)

A condition known as familial *hypercholesterolemia* is found in one of 500 children, which is a pretty high average and worthy of parental awareness. Left untreated, 23% of men with the condition will experience fatal coronary events by age 50. One in five hundred might seem like pretty fair odds, but to someone whose child is affected those odds were not good enough. The actual complete name of this disease is *Heterozygous familial hypercholesterolemia* (or HeFH). A study led by Dr. Evan Stein of *Medical Research Laboratories of* Highland Heights, Kentucky, was "the largest and longest placebo-controlled trial of any lipid-lowering drug in an adolescent population."

## SUMMARY

The combined professional advice would suggest that it would certainly make sense to know your children's inherited heart risk profile as well as their cholesterol and environmental influences. The earlier the better, when measures by *natural means* can be implemented to protect a child from developing heart disease. If many of these markers and mechanisms are found to be out of line, what better time to deal with them? As you are now aware, heart disease diagnosed in later years had been lying like a tiger ready to strike for a very long time. The length and quality of these youngster's lives will be increased if more is done to intervene preventively early in the process.

Many of our "indestructible" young people are consuming fast food diets overloaded with *trans and saturated fats*. They are smoking and engaged in too little exercise. Even if these contributing forces set the course of what might happen in midlife (as the doctor Nissen has suggested), the victims would still be in their prime.

# Chapter 6

# Argument *for*
# *Earlier Drug Intervention*

Is it counter-productive for physicians to spend as much time trying to get patients to reduce high cholesterol counts through diet and exercise as has been the accepted practice? Would there be added health benefit for the patient if doctors prescribed drugs sooner rather than later? Is it possible that the amount of advancement of atherosclerosis and additional occlusion during the wait and watch period would be more harmful than any risk from prescribing the drug to a qualified candidate in the first place? In fact, the latest research from the leaders in the scientific community leans strongly in this direction. More often than not, patients with all good intentions lose a minimal amount of weight and their cholesterol count continues to remain at a dangerously high level.

**After a year or two of attempts to reduce cholesterol naturally, the "trial and error" experiment may possibly have permitted increased arterial damage.**

In the vast majority of cases, without drug benefit these patients, sadly, do not meet their ideal goals and consequently remain anxious and frustrated. In some borderline and moderate cases the natural approach has worked quite well, however in too many other cases it has been a recipe for extension of patient risk. There is a point of diminishing returns; would it not be prudent to move to cholesterol therapy *sooner rather than later?* The time to talk about whether or not the particular patient would remain on the drug would be a year or two later when and if they reduced the desired 50 lbs. *and* their cholesterol dropped to 200 from a previous 298. The patient has often been denied therapy much too long, and we must ask if there was a monetary reason for a provider to delay treatment. I knew one lady with a total cholesterol of 275 and an LDL of 156 who was not prescribed medication for over two years and efforts to bring her levels down *naturally* proved feeble at best. You might know someone with a similar story. What has been the justification? It cannot be just the efficacy *(safety)* factor because statin therapy safety is very well established. At the first sign of a problem the doctor would take the patient off the medication. Might it be plausible that a major insurance company or HMO would save millions if for example, 50,000 adult patients across the country were encouraged to delay going on expensive cholesterol medication for just one or two years? Let's do the math: at an approximate $67.00 average medication cost to the insurance company, would this provider not save $3,350,000 dollars per month, amounting to $80,400,000 over two years?

*New Guidelines:* In early 2001, the guidelines for cholesterol were finally lowered, thereby including thousands more who would benefit from drug therapy.

According to the newly recommended guidelines, approximately 23 million more patients should be administered cholesterol medications than currently are. Would new lower guidelines alter you or someone you know from a *borderline at-risk* status into a more *at-risk* category? Now, after more than ten years of use of the statin drugs, follow up studies have shown so many important surprising health benefits for the patient that go beyond the drug's originally recognized purpose.

## THE IMPRESSIVE NEWLY-DISCOVERED BENEFITS OF STATIN THERAPY

Doctor Ikuo Yokoyama and his colleagues of Japan were studying whether or not cholesterol affects the ability of arteries to expand and retract in a function known as *myocardial vasodilation* (MVD). For the purpose of the study the criteria called for administering cholesterol-lowering drugs not only to those patients *with known coronary artery disease* but also specifically to subjects who had *neither heart disease nor* elevated cholesterol. The two subsets of patients would be evaluated for their state of *vasodilation* over one year. At the end of the study, both groups had shown significant results in improvement in MVD because of statin therapy. Cholesterol-lowering drugs have now actually demonstrated an ability to aid in the *preservation of arterial health by countering* impaired myocardial vasodilation, (hardened inflexible arteries).

In addition to earlier findings that statins reduced heart attacks, strokes and overall mortality, the following previously unrealized potential lifesaving benefits are now being recognized. They are:

> ▶ The drug's ability to help regulate better *bone health*.
> ▶ The drug's ability to regress *hardening of the arteries, improving vasodilation*.
> ▶ The drug's ability to mediate against *inflammation*.

The following findings will prove to be of major encouragement to anyone prescribed cholesterol-lowering drugs. At the 2001 Sessions of *The American Heart Association*, the results of a *Simvastatin* study substantiated this drug's ability...

**TO NOT ONLY INHIBIT THE PROGRESSION OF SUSCEPTIBLE, "VULNERABLE" ARTERIAL PLAQUE, BUT ALSO TO DECREASE THE ACTUAL SIZE OF EXISTING ATHEROSCLEROTIC PLAQUE.**

Dr. Roberto Coti, M.D. from the *Mount Sinai School of Medicine* in New York City, reported not only a predictable 30-35% decrease in cardiovascular events as a result of a total and LDL cholesterol reduction but also cited a marked reduction in existing plaque formation. Researchers and scientists search for any therapy that brings *even a small amount of plaque regression*. That is the reason there was so much excitement when the newly discovered benefits of statin therapy were announced.

*Actual regression of atherosclerotic lesions (plaques) in both the thoracic aorta (main coronary artery) and the carotid (neck) arteries was discovered.* **There was also a reported 8% significant <u>decrease</u> in the thickness of the wall of the *aorta* at the end of one year's time, and a 7% plaque reduction in the carotid arteries found at the end of two years. Exciting, encouraging news.**

*The increase in lumen space, (open channel in the artery) had become enlarged due to a <u>decrease</u> in the thickness of the vessel wall. The final result was a significant reduction in both aortic and carotid lesions .*

Any patient on statin therapy for high cholesterol should be encouraged by this valuable information. Here is why.

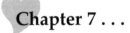 Chapter 7 . . .

# *Plaques*
# *that Burst like Fireworks*

Almost all of us, as time goes on, will develop a certain amount of plaque in our arteries and why one person dislodges the plaque and another does not has been an unanswered question until now.

> **Vulnerable plaque is <u>one of the most</u> important determining factors as to which plaque is most prone to rupture, resulting in the heart attack or stroke.**

A report concerning this particular issue was offered at the 72nd Scientific Sessions of the *American Heart Association* in 11/1999 in a tribute to Dr. Russell Ross, a man often referred to as the *"founder of contemporary vascular biology."* Dr. Russell Ross like most pioneers sailed his own course far ahead of his time.

Dr. Ross was the first to explore the
possibility that atherosclerosis, rather than being of
a degenerative process is actually the result of an
inflammatory one. A concept contrary to the theory
that had been previously accepted as gospel.

The types of plaques (their characterization, diagnosis
and treatment) were discussed in the presentation. M.D.s
Deborah Gershon and Valentin Fuster (former President
of the American Heart Association) described the most
dangerous form as ... "vulnerable plaque."

*Vulnerable plaque would be the plaque most likely to*
*rupture and produce an acute coronary consequence.*

Different plaque types and what would make them
more likely to explode or rupture have now been identified by their particular composition in their various stages
of development. A process that becomes hastened under
certain inflammatory conditions. In a paper written by
AHA members assigned to a committee reporting on the
pathophysiology (physical construction) of Coronary Artery Calcification, members *Wexler, Brundage, Fuster,
Rumberger, Crouse* and others on the team actually identified five phases of coronary plaques, from their early
beginnings as "fatty streaks" to eventual advanced lesion
and rupture.

> *"Indeed, recently it has become apparent that arteriographically mild coronary lesions may undergo significant progression to severe stenosis or total occlusion over a period of a few months."*

In other words, what might appear to be a small seemingly "mild plaque" or a "fatty streak" has the growth potential to accelerate at any time. Presumably here would lie one possible answer to a question that has troubled medicine for years, and particularly, since the wide use of treadmills and angiograms. The question of how someone could pass a treadmill or an angiogram catherization with flying colors and a few weeks or a few months later have a heart attack or die of plaque disruption remained unanswered until now.

## —VITAL INFORMATION—
## ONE OF THE MAJOR CAUSES
## OF HEART ATTACK

James J. Stec, BS, a research scientist at *the Institute for Prevention of Cardiovascular Disease,* along with Geoffrey H. Tofler, MBBS Associate Professor of Medicine at *Harvard Medical School,* in addressing the vulnerability of plaques, said:

*" physiologic forces that are rapidly generated by external triggers may acutely lead to plaque disruption and thrombosis, "*

in what the authors call, *"The final pathway of most myocardial infarctions"* (heart attacks). These physiologic forces the doctor is referring to are the ones you and I are reviewing.

# INTRAVASCULAR ULTRASOUND
# DEFINES PLAQUE TYPE

*Intravascular Ultrasound* (IVUS) procedures can now permit doctors to examine plaque construction and composition within the actual artery. For this purpose this newer technology is more effective than *angiography* which, since it's introduction has been used successfully as the "gold standard" in determining stenosis (blockage) size. However, like all technology it too has had it's limitations. In contrast to angiogram, IVUS permits the physician for the first time to observe plaque in its various constructive or destructive stages of development. *Plaques are not all alike and a small plaque in a short period of time can rapidly progress in size to the stage where its rupture could certainly be fatal to the patient.* All the while, an angiogram might have concluded that this same patient was not at risk as the catherization only observed a small unobtrusive sized lesion.

> **THE TYPE OF PLAQUE IS MORE INDICATIVE OF A POTENTIAL RUPTURE THAN EVEN THE ANGIOGRAM'S SIZE EVALUATION.**

The classifications are *soft plaque, hard plaque* and *vulnerable plaque*. The descriptive words "stable" and "unstable" are often used to describe the different plaques. Angiograms, according to the doctor, can detect a blockage as small as 20-30%. Most doctors observing these small lesions would assume them to be mostly insignificant. From the results of ultrasound examination, Dr. Nissen concluded that **a relatively small blockage could actually be holding a large threatening plaque within the apparently harmless stenosis.** Heretofore, the physician and the patient might have been elated upon learning that the small blockages found during their angiogram were minor and therefore not of major concern. According to Dr. Nissen's findings, these patients would not necessarily be out of the woods. The doctor found two particular categorical definitions of plaques.

1. *The first one, he explains, presents with a large lipid core and a thin fibrous cap. He instructs that this type is vulnerable to rupture.*

2. *The second type has less of a lipid core but a thicker cap and appears even more vulnerable to rupture.*

A meta-analysis report appeared in the *South Dakota Journal of Medicine.*

> **The report informed us that 68% of most acute coronary events actually strike in arteries which have even LESS than a 50% stenosis. ONLY 14% take place in stenotic lesions within arteries that have occlusion greater than 70%.**

According to these findings, you can take little comfort in learning you have very small lesions even though everyone around you might be jumping up and down and *high-fiving* you from the angiogram result. Additional supportive trials have found that these smaller blockages were built with *fatty plaque* and can actually dislodge and rupture more easily than the major sized **harder plaque** composition that everyone has been afraid of. There is some good news, and that is that *statin* drugs (like Zocor) have proved, in recently completed long-term studies, to afford protection by inhibiting growth of fatty deposits within the actual blockages. The studies have also observed actual **retardation** of *existing* plaque.

## HOW IMPORTANT IS THIS NEW PLAQUE INFORMATION FOR THE PATIENT?

**It is not only significant but it is one of the most important, up-to-date breakthroughs in understanding how plaques can burst, or explode in the causation of heart attacks.**

Plaque stabilization is indeed complicated by *inflammatory factors* as well as other external triggers. In just the past few years cardiology has advanced light years in knowledge including coming to an understanding of how such things as smooth cell proliferation, *T-cells, cytokines, macrophages,* and *leukocytes* damage artery walls. **Each of us has probably experienced having a blood-rich infected sore at one time or another. We can recall how profusely the scab bled when it was picked or became dislodged.** This is a very simple illustration of how inflammation within a plaque or **underlying the base** of the plaque festers, eventually bursting, into hemorrhage.

There is great risk of bleeding from these lipid-rich plaques. This condition can obviously translate into a heart attack. Is there anything you or I as patients can do to determine if inflammation is active in our systems? One thing you can do is to insist on a hi-sensitivity CRP blood test. If significant inflammation is in progress in your body this test would indicate its presence. As I explained earlier, another advantage to taking daily aspirin is that it was found in the Physician's Health Study that the compound reduces inflammation by 55.7%. As important as this protection is, the real need is to identify and mediate the actual cause of inflammation. Another is to be sure to include adequate antioxidants to counter the damage of destructive free radicals, and of course work to maintain optimal cholesterol, particularly LDL levels. If significant inflammation is in progress a CRP test should indicate its presence. There is great need to identify and mediate the actual cause of the inflammation. Remember, statin drugs do fight inflammation, and inflammation at the artery wall beneath a plaque offers a very unstable base that is subject to displacement. CRP has been mentioned earlier. Later in this chapter will be a detailed explanation of this very important risk factor.

**Dr. Valentin Fuster,** currently with the Mount Siani Medical Center in New York, is using a different approach; *hi-sensitivity MRI* (with agent) in studies to identify plaques in their various stages, and especially those that are most apt to rupture. It may take five years before this procedure is available to the general public, but the technology is in place. This is being touted as the one overall evaluation that will soon offer the cardiologist a "one stop" evaluation. MRI is being tested currently in several hospital medical studies that have shown this non-invasive technology able to record with 75% accuracy blockages in the coronary arteries for minor plaques and 89% for the more seriously developed larger lesions. More work is still needed to bring this technology to the current standard of the invasive, but currently more accurate, angiogram evaluation. The following chapter offers a *fictional* account to illustrate how the new preventive approach might interpret familial history and support earlier intervention to identify the at-risk patient. A process that would utilize the new methodologies to diagnose and treat. This imagined scenario probably isn't too far a stretch.

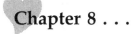

# Chapter 8 . . .

# *Fictional Reality,*
## *applying the* New Information

Strictly for the purpose of illustration, consider a patient with an undiagnosed dysfunction such as high *fibrinogen* (a recently emerging <u>serious</u> risk concern). This factor can become complicated by a situation as apparently innocent, but significant (as we will see), as living in an extremely cold area of the country. Now besides having this high fibrinogen and living in a severe cold climate, this same *fictional* person also smokes (high fibrinogen levels are very often found among smokers). This patient also has an undiscovered severely dysfunctional *inherited* LP (a) gene and had also recorded an elevated 135 LDL cholesterol on his last physical. A level which *by itself* may <u>not</u> have particularly alarmed the physician. If another fact be known, there had been a family history of very low HDL cholesterol blamed on the father's side. In this hypothetical case, it is entirely possible (based on the science) that cold weather, along with the **combination** of the inherited and acquired dysfunctions...

1. LP (a) (inherited gene)
2. fibrinogen (acquired/inherited)
3. smoking (acquired risk)
4. low HDL (inherited)

...would turn out to be the same *individual undetected causes* that had previously claimed the lives of this subject's immediate relatives before him and now would hasten his own death. If the information being presented here had been available to this patient and his physician, these "hidden" factors would **not** have remained hidden and could have been treated.

Now if the same combination of *undetected and unrealized* risk factors prematurely claimed the life of this unsuspecting subject, would the commonly accepted explanation be that his demise had been caused by something unavoidable? Would his be just another case filed and dismissed under the umbrella of "heredity?"

While heredity, in a broad sense would have been partly culpable, patients like our subject have been suffering heart attacks and strokes and have left this world much too early because of unidentified *hidden* risk factors. It doesn't have to be that way any longer if the advice of the leading edge scientists, researchers and physicians is heeded. You are becoming the patient who understands the need for proper evaluation.

Among the markers which we will study together are homocysteine, inflammation and its various causes, bacterial/viral infections and inherited genetic predisposition, particularly in relationship to lipid (cholesterol) management. Heart disease is the number one killer. Nothing, absolutely nothing that is available in diagnostics should be overlooked or ignored. As the evidence will continue to show, it is not at all unusual to find *more than one inherited risk factor* in a given individual's risk profile. With a physician now able for the first time to look at the results of the new diagnostics in this individualized manner, the patient will no doubt benefit. How many doctors are regularly testing for these novel traits in diagnosing their patient's risk evaluations? **HOW MANY OF THESE TESTS ARE PERFORMED INVESTIGATIVELY LONG BEFORE THE INDIVIDUAL EVER GAINS THE UNENVIABLE TITLE OF "HEART DISEASE PATIENT"?** Is it not becoming obvious why *heredity as the overall cause can no longer serve to explain away such cardiovascular events?* One can inherit heart disease mechanisms, but it is not a given that the patient need automatically succumb to heart disease.

## FOR THE RECORD

*Incidentally, for the record, in regard to the fictional illustration we used—yes, fibrinogen definitely becomes elevated among smokers. The study in N. ENGL J. MED. Vol. 311/8, 1984, as well as other studies, showed that, in fact fibrinogen does reach higher levels in cold weather.* A later chapter addresses this *fibrinogen* risk factor which by itself, according to a 1966 *Benderly* study published in *Arteriosclerosis, Thrombosis and Vascular Biology,* can increase one's risk of heart attack as much as 85%! To recap: a combination of the risk factor of smoking, aggravated by very cold weather and inactivity (particularly during the winter months) could in fact increase fibrinogen level and complicate one's risk of heart disease and cardiac death. *For the record,* it is a fact that heart attacks do increase during December and January of each year and lessen in warmer months. A study originating in France analyzed and tracked some 138,602 people who had died in the years 1992-1996. The results show that throughout the five years of the study, death from heart disease increased and peaked during each winter. In January the death rate *was 20% higher* than the average month. In contrast, August deaths were actually down 15%. Do these statistics imply that fibrinogen's elevated response to cold weather is the singular cause of this increased death rate sighted in the studies? Certainly not, but interestingly, this particular study did come to its conclusions after discounting all other causes. The *Scottish Heart Health Study* (among others) determined that fibrinogen is a factor to be considered when evaluating a patient's family history of premature heart disease. Imagine, **if patients like our fictional one or his relatives had lived today and their particular inflammatory and inherited risk factors had been identified through the available diagnostics. Is it not feasible that the early discovery and treatment** of these risks could possibly have prompted the removal of their names from an early departure list? It is becoming apparent that elevated fibrinogen, along with the other *hidden causes* which we will study, have been contributing causes of premature death for a very long, long time. You are now becoming aware of it, and hopefully your doctor is keeping up with the newest scientific findings. For the first time, the *American Heart Association* has identified high fibrinogen as an independent risk factor comparable to cholesterol and smoking. This organization has recommended that doctors now consider evaluating certain patients for high levels. Of five individuals whom the author had interviewed and whose doctors agreed to evaluate fibrinogen, three (including the author) had scores beyond the top 85% risk range according to Benderly's 1966 study. You will be presented many other studies that basically agree on the importance of identifying and containing this risk factor. These same individuals who agreed to be tested were also found to have additional risk factors in their profiles and two had earlier suffered *first heart attacks.*

> **How would this newer, conscientious preventive approach affect the overall numbers of heart disease and premature death in this country within the next 15 or 20 years if monitoring, identifying and treating all of the individual dysfunctions were the goal of all primary physicians and cardiologists?**

The cost of managing health care for heart disease patients is 60 billion dollars each year!

# Chapter 9 . . .

# *an* *Author's Journey*

B efore exploring many of the additional "silent" risk factors including *fibrinogen,* this would probably be as good a time as any to explain why I became so involved with this subject, and why I felt it necessary to become entrenched in the related research. I had actually begun writing the book earlier but after quite unexpectedly stumbling upon a crisis in my own life, in finding an extremely high fibrinogen and calcification score, I had little choice but to become more involved. *It was not a motivation I had wished for.* I had not desired to reveal personal health details, but it became apparent that not sharing them would do a disservice to the information and ultimately the reader. If I were you, I would want to see what the actual results are when all this knowledge is applied. I have come to this information after just about five years of exploration. *It is not my information* — it is the work of hundreds of dedicated scientific teams guided by leading researchers, scientists and physicians. It will now become your information. As history has taught us, the research community is usually 15-20 years ahead of the mainstream practicing office. It is after all, the research community that discovers and proves or disproves the information that the physicians will follow in their daily practice. When a patient finds they have a potentially dangerous medical problem and are unable to locate a physician familiar with the malady at the time and how to evaluate or rectify it, the patient unfortunately is put at great disadvantage. You have two choices: to live in ignorance and be a victim, or become your own researcher and hopefully by acquiring knowledge, remain ahead of the curve. No one obviously will have the vested interest you would have as the patient. Let's begin and I will try to make it entertaining. Medical information can make for very dry reading.

## THE LONG AND WINDING ROAD

Several years ago I read a considerable amount of information about a new breakthrough ultra-fast CT scan that could detect the amount and location of calcification throughout the coronary arteries. The technology was relatively new and was called EBCT (electron beam computed tomography). A technology capable of evaluating what might be in progression in even a asymptomatic (without symptom) patient's coronary arterial system. Isn't this what we had been waiting for—a non-invasive look at what is taking place internally? And so it began. I had been to too many funerals of friends through the years—as perhaps you have also—friends who had met an early demise from a heart attack without prior warning. On this occasion, two longtime friends were coming to town from the Pacific Northwest. Together they must have actually conspired to break every cardinal rule for maintaining proper health, diet and exercise ever written! These guys were definite candidates for the scan, and my intention was to do what I thought would be a good thing, helping them each avoid a heart attack. I would take them to UCLA for the 5-minute *look-see!* I had no plans to include myself in this endeavor. A small problem immediately arose: if I wasn't going to have the scan, they weren't either. Nothing insurmountable...in the end, all three of us took the scan. My two friends went through the test basically unscathed (although one had a somewhat elevated score and a cholesterol-lowering medication was in order, even though his cholesterol was a little over 200). It was MY score that registered "tilt," come and get me! Is there a doctor in the house and did I hear someone say, "Dead Man Walking?" Me and my big ideas. Had I needed this test? Do you need this test? All traditional indications would have precluded me as a patient who would benefit from the scan. I think we could safely have assumed that 95% of doctors in 1998 would have looked at my collective cholesterol readings, thallium treadmill scores and dietary habits and concluded that this patient should save the money. But to give you an idea of just how high the score actually was, it is important to realize first that according to the Mayo Clinic's reference scale as established for the *Imatron* EBCT scan, 400 would be considered a *severe* score. **My first score was recorded at 1770. Four and a half times or 450% beyond severe!** This goes to the point that if doctors are only concerned with cholesterol as a means of determining his or her "at risk" heart attack or stroke patients, they could be seriously missing the mark. It was a few days after having the scans that the reporting doctor called to relay the results. I remember at the beginning of our conversation (before the caller could actually do more than identify himself), my asking how my friends had done on the scan. "Well," said the doctor, "your friends did quite well, it is you we are concerned with." Me? "No way, you guys made an error, I think you have my buddy's films confused with mine." I'm the one who never had a cholesterol score higher than 200, who hadn't eaten an egg in 12 years (substituting egg beaters), who has only drunk nonfat milk and eaten low-fat dairy products for 25 years. I am also the guy who doesn't smoke, and who a couple of months before had passed a yearly nuclear treadmill with honors! Ahh! "Doc, I think I know what went wrong. You see there were three of us who took the scan back to back, and someone tracking the three probably got the sequence messed up. It happens, right?" Now I was thinking that if there had been a mistake as to whose chart it was, I would have a real dilemma on my hands. How the hell am I going to break the bad news to one of these two friends whom I had convinced to take the scan? All of these thoughts were going through my mind in a nanosecond.

## THE OLD GOOD NEWS/BAD NEWS SCENARIO

The good news for me would be that the radiologist had given me the wrong score and I had since learned I was as healthy as a horse! The bad news—alas, "one of you guys is destined for a heart attack!" But no, there was no mistake—the extreme score of 1770 belonged to yours truly. What proved amazing to me was to later learn that four cardiologists, whom I have since spoken to either socially or in an interview situation, have denied the need for the scan in spite of all the information in the medical journals confirming its probative ability. What seemed ludicrous was that at the same time they were making this denial they readily admitted that calcification (which is what the scan measures) is indeed what eventually causes blockages and classic "hardening of the arteries." The idea did cross my suspicious mind that this technology could alert the patient years before they would become another angioplasty or open-heart case. The person would learn the information (as did I) while there was still ample time to initiate drug therapy or dietary changes, and at the very least alert the physician to do further diagnostic exploration. The EBCT does not record the size of a blockage, except when used as a non-invasive (EBA) angiogram. EBCT does however record the building blocks of calcification and the remodeling that precedes actual stenosis or "blockage." If doctors are looking at the end result of a scan expecting to find a one-to-one correlation between calcium score and actual blockage for their interpretation they would probably not realize the true essence of this technology. It is a valuable tool to alert both the physician and the patient to implement therapy to avoid the greater consequence. How then would this information and identification of calcification affect the revenue of the physician or surgeon's office? Fluoride in the drinking water eliminated a need for a whole lot of dental work and disrupted a significant revenue stream for dentistry. *Glucosomine* and *chondroitin sulfate* (two natural healing substances) are bringing relief to thousands of osteo arthritis patients. MSM (methyl-sulfonyl-methane) for rheumatoid sufferers is permitting many patients to toss their prescriptions of *methotrexate, prednisone, naprosyn* and other severe drugs. Not meaning disrespect, what effect would the EBCT scanner have on a surgeon or cardiologist's revenue stream? Four years ago everyone seemed to be looking at cholesterol as the only reason for this high amount of calcification. I was not persuaded, as I remembered the information that **50% of heart attacks occur among people with normal cholesterol.** A quote you will find repeated, but does not reappear by accident. As a matter of fact, many of the people I had known or heard of through the years who had heart attacks had "normal" cholesterol levels. And so my research into the results of close to 1,000 clinical studies research papers and related articles on heart disease began. It quickly became obvious that none of the doctors **I initially consulted had at that time any interest in exploring inflammatory or individual inherited risk factors;** they seemed only to direct therapy at the cholesterol level. I did not choose the role of researcher, it was chosen for me, by virtue of the fact that I had to decide whether I would become a victim or an advocate.

One thing became obvious, and that was that if the calcification continued accumulating with the cause not identified (as high as the risk already was for a heart attack or stroke) the already high bar would be grossly raised even higher. John Rumberger M.D., Ph.D., at the time with the *Mayo Clinic* in Rochester, among his other responsibilities was setting the guidelines for coronary calcification risk assessment as well as educating physicians in practical interpretation of EBCT technology. Most people would have the single scan and probably then be prescribed one of the statin drugs, and they or their physicians would not see a need for retesting. Hundreds if not thousands of patients who had presented with far less calcification than I, have been scheduled for follow-up thallium treadmills, and those who could not perform satisfactorily were given angiogram evaluations resulting in angioplasties or open-heart surgery. *I was convinced that my negative result would not ultimately be determined to have been the result of choles-*

*terol. I was intent upon identifying the cause(s) for my high score as much from a clinical research standpoint as from an individual health search.* In order to do this, I believed it would be necessary to monitor my progress over time and submit to additional follow-up screenings in this effort. I consulted two cardiologists during this period, but they seemed not to want to move beyond cholesterol management supported by annual treadmill exams. They had little interest in looking elsewhere. You can imagine how encouraged I was to later meet two local physicians who would agree with my approach.

My EBCT score, originally 1,770, would continue to increase, progressing to 2,680 (as recorded on the same machine and evaluated by the same radiologist) over the next three years before fibrinogen and homocysteine, the ultimate contributing forces, would finally be identified and arrested. If you recall, 400 was the threshold for scores considered severe.

*Incidentally, during this entire period my cholesterol profile was maintained through combination therapy with a total cholesterol 157, LDL 77, triglycerides 72 and HDL 66.* There was no other option than to get personally entrenched in this search, which, as we will share, would lead far beyond cholesterol. Hopefully, what you learn will benefit you or someone close to you. The author is merely the recipient and the conduit of the work of leading researchers and scientists from all over the world. Perhaps I may claim the application of the science, but the knowledge comes from the dedicated pioneers in the research community who always seem to be years ahead of the traditional practicing office. It is the research community whose dedication defies all accepted protocol and eventually establishes new standards for physicians to follow. It is my desire that my expense and effort in searching for answers will help you better address the newer cardiovascular diagnostics and treatment in discussions with your doctor about you and your family's healthcare.

Consider this: the *American Heart Association* announced that the Imatron Ultra-Fast CT scan is ten times more effective than cholesterol readings in predicting individuals heading for heart attacks. In another release in the journal *Cardiology* in 1997, it was announced that the scan was 97% accurate in diagnosing calcification in asymptomatic patients (exhibiting no symptoms). These are amazing statistics when you consider the body of evidence in favor of the scan originating from such reliable sources. Why then are insurance companies and HMO's still not funding this test as a diagnostic tool? Incidentally, it is the same technology that is now used in the "Full Body" scan you might have read about. One fortuitous caveat is that the patient may pay the $390 themselves and order the coronary scan without a prescription as I did. Hopefully, you will not have the same results. That 5-minute, painless and non-invasive scan might well have saved my life or at least helped me avoid a heart attack. The follow-up medical advice was that I keep my cholesterol in check. My cholesterol had never been a problem and now it was exemplary, so now what?

The question came to mind, early in the research, of why one patient with a high total cholesterol of 255 or higher and an associated high LDL of 145 and HDL of 40, would present with little or no calcification, while another patient with total C of 197, an LDL of 110 and an HDL of 45 would still have <u>extensive calcification</u>?

> **It soon became obvious, that any doctor not explor-
> ing their patient's markers for *inflammatory or
> inherited* factors would miss many opportunities to
> avoid their patient's future heart attack or stroke.**

Much of the information that is being presented to you I
have actually applied in search of my own contributing
risk factors to learn what would be required to stabilize
the calcification process, and what might be involved in
beginning actual reversal. A word to the wise: a high
calcification score should encourage you to seek your
doctor's intervention and advice. A treadmill may be what
he or she would advise for the next step in determining
the best course of action.

    **"Hello, Mr. Cardiologist; I think I need to have a
new thallium treadmill evaluation."** I explained that
I had just learned that I was the proud possessor of
enough heavy- duty calcification lodged in my arteries to build another LA freeway. "How do you know
that?" asked the doctor. "I had a EBCT scan at UCLA."
"Well," said the doctor, "I think the test is bogus."
Really? Bogus? Are you saying the millions of dollars the major universities and respected hospitals
all over the world are investing in the EBCT scanner
at a cost of 2.5 million dollars apiece is bogus? (UCLA
has three, as does the Mayo Clinic). The doctor re-
plied, "I have stock in the company, and it's going to
make a lot of money, but I think the procedures we
have in place, angiograms and treadmills, do a better
job." I asked him if there was any doubt that calcifi-

cation was the cornerstone in the construction of plaque and eventual blockages in the progression of heart disease. "Yes" was the answer, and so I asked a naive patient's question: "Well, excuse me, but if calcification is at the core of the problem then why wouldn't a patient and the physician want to detect it at the earliest possible time?" Doctor's response; "That is what the treadmill and the angiogram are for." I couldn't help thinking I was the straight man in a *Laurel and Hardy* routine! But isn't that what we want to avoid, *Ollie*, the need for an angiogram or open-heart surgery in the first place? Wouldn't it be more advantageous to identify the problem long before the treadmill finds it? Discovering advanced artherosclerosis on the treadmill, isn't that just a little late?

"All I know" said the doctor, "is that we are going to do as many angiograms with or without the CT scan. Let's go ahead and see what we learn from the treadmill."

Well the good news was that I passed beautifully, as I had earlier, and I was understandably relieved. It could have been a much different story. The doctors (based on the degree of calcification already ascertained) could have been scheduling me for a subsequent angiogram and possibly even open-heart surgery. The problem apparently was discovered before significant blockages or "remodeling" had impeded the blood flow to an appreciable degree. Still, there could be no denying the amount of calcification present. My excitement waned a bit, however, when I later learned that passing a treadmill isn't conclusive proof of not having sizable blockages. You should be aware that in fact the information is that it is not uncommon for stenosis of *70-75% to go undetected even by the nuclear treadmill.* That sounded like a pretty large obstruction that could slip through the diagnostic net. This would be <u>one</u> explanation of why people can have excellent treadmills and two days or a few months later experience a massive heart attack, as a hemorrhage or a portion of plaque lodges against an already compromised 65-75% stenosis. The standard advice I was given was to come back in a year and repeat this wonderful process. The advice reminded me of a car transmission TV ad I had seen some time earlier: "Pay now, or pay later." In other words, we are going to get your butt one way or another, it's just a matter of time. If you didn't fall off the treadmill the first time, perhaps you would the following year, and then the physician would know *exactly* what to do. Here would be the intervention. Here would come the angioplasty or the open-heart surgery. Here would come the $55,000 surgery bill, or the angioplasty bill for $5600 to $10,000. **Make no mistake, these procedures are incredible advancements and there is no doubt about it, they do save lives. Only a fool would deny that.** The men and women who would intervene on your and my behalf are *miracle workers.* If anyone ever gets to the point that they need one of these procedures, they should thank their lucky stars that the practitioners who administer these lifesaving procedures are available. But with all due respect, isn't the object **TO AVOID NEEDING A MIRACLE** at all?

## CAUSE AND EFFECT

Just as importantly, these procedures only correct the problem temporarily. **Many open-heart surgeries will have**

**to be repeated within a few years if the source of the problem that got you under the surgeon's knife in the first place wasn't identified and eliminated.** And you know what? Unless the right blood tests are done and a complete evaluation performed, these contributing factors we are discussing will be back at work continuing their destructive course. When an open-heart surgery is performed, smaller vessels are used to replace the larger natural arteries where the source of the problem originated. **These smaller vessels can occlude much sooner because they have a smaller lumen (open channel) capacity than the patient's larger, normal arteries which took a lifetime to close.** Additional angioplasties may have to be done as *re-stenosis* causes re-closure of the affected artery. Recently science has provided surgeons the ability to radiate the immediate area of an angioplasty as stents (metal sleeves) are inserted to keep arteries open permanently.

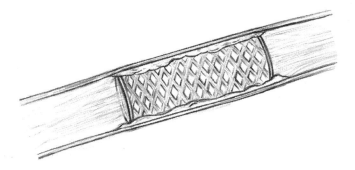

Fig 2: Metal stent

The body's natural repair mechanisms often overcompensate in their healing process, building repair tissue at the site which may become scar tissue, thereby advancing re-stenosis (blocking) of the artery. One other advancement currently being used is the application of a medicated coating on stents that inhibits secondary occlusion (re-stenosis). All we are discussing is the destructive process from early **cause to final effect**. The final effect however, would be a non-issue if the actual cause or causes could be discovered early on. **Without the scan, could anyone know their degree of calcification and how it might be contributing to their risk profile?** The information bears repeating: The American Heart Association has published studies that have concluded the scan is **"95% accurate in detecting future heart attacks among asymptomatic people."** You would think insurance companies would be clamoring at the possibility of detecting and averting disease at the earliest possible point in time. The EBCT "full body" scan does just that. There is a difference in the low amount of radiation one is exposed to during the EBCT as opposed to spiral imaging, which is another type of scanning. Dr. Rumberger, the world authority on EBCT, explains that living in Los Angeles probably exposes one to a measure of radiation of 300 Rads per day. The coronary scan exposes one to 100 Rads.

## PHASE TWO

In actuality, what did all this mean, and what could I expect? I should at this point tell you that this first scan was in 1998, and since then much of the monolithic approach to heart disease has been changing, thanks to the advancement of the work of pioneering doctors like William Castelli of the *Framingham Heart Study*, and other leading doctors like Robert Superko, Ronald Krauss of the *Berkeley Heartlab*, Dr. Valentin Fuster; former President of

*The American Heart Association*, and doctors Paul Ridker, of *Harvard Medical and Brigham Women's hospital*, Michael Gaziano (also with *Harvard*), Michael Miller of the *University of Maryland*, Dr. Steven Nissen, *Cleveland Clinic Foundation*, John Rumberger with the *Ohio State University*, Dr. Rene Malinow of *Oregon State University* and Antonio Gotto from *Cornell Medical Center*. The list of pioneers of inherited and environmental factors must include, in particular, three gentlemen, two of whose early work in the 1950's and 60's built a foundation for much of what has since been developed at the *Lawrence Berkeley National Laboratory* in regard to VLDL (very low density lipoproteins), IDL (intermediate dense lipoprotein) and the sub-classification (further breakdown) of both *low density (LDL) and high density (HDL) lipoproteins*. Frank Lindgren and the former Director of Molecular Medicine, John Gofman, established the basis for what Berkeley HeartLab's Ronald Krauss M.D. and Robert Superko M.D., FACC, have brought to fruition: namely, the development of diagnostic tests that can now identify previously undetected dysfunctions. The third gentlemen who should be recognized for his pioneering effort is **Dr. Russell Ross (now deceased) from the University of Washington, whose early work in identifying the inflammatory factors has proven to be absolutely visionary.** Much of the new science will be presented in this book as a protective source of material for you to discuss with your physician under the category of *Preventive Cardiology*. In the meantime, after learning of the EBCT result, I consulted with 2 cardiologists and a primary physician in Southern California. At the time, no one seemed intimately familiar with the inflammatory or inherited factors you and I are discussing, and had little interest in going beyond cholesterol as the culprit. I was told to keep my cholesterol in check, to shed a few pounds and play a little more golf. Well, to begin with, I don't play golf, so that advice fell on a deaf ear. The second useless piece of advice was that stress was a big no-no, and not to worry! While any patient is concentrating on *not* getting stressed, they become *more* stressed at the very prospect of going under the knife. All the while, the kind physician is doing his or her best to quiet their patient's concerns. As a cardiologist told a friend of mine, "remember, this is what we do every day; we operate on patients with heart problems! It has become pretty routine surgery." Pretty routine?

# Chapter 10

# *There are no*
# *Routine Surgeries*

Routine? What the hell is "routine" about being cut open like a chicken from stem to stern? What's routine about letting a stranger saw your breastbone in two and having your ribs pulled apart by a miniature set of *Jaws of Life*? What is routine about having a dilating IV dispensing a serious drug into your veins that could possibly cause heart *fibrillation* or *anaphylactic* shock? What is routine about having a machine breathe for you while you lie somewhere between life and death? The more we see accounts of "life after death" given by the patient who died on the operating table later to be resuscitated, the more we realize how many things do go wrong during those *"routine surgeries."* There have been more than thirteen million such cases reported—but we certainly don't have to rely on this form of record keeping when there are scientific and legitimate sources that speak to the problem. So, what would be routine about a year's recovery, with coumadin running through your veins, or the calculated risk of dying on the operating table, or having a post surgery heart attack, or **the one to five percent risk of a major stroke because of displaced or unstable plaque?** The heart and lung machine is attached at the *aorta*, which is the largest artery involved in the procedure—and, as a matter of fact, the largest artery in the body. It is here where a good deal of plaque disruption occurs, particularly among patients who have had significant calcification present in the aorta. **The successful treadmill gave me some hope that if I could find a physician who would co-partner with me in an effort to explore beyond the cholesterol, I might be able to halt the calcification process and hopefully begin to regress some of the high score. As you can imagine, finding someone who was aware of the new mechanisms five years ago was not an easy task.** There will be another chapter heading called *Part Two of the Author's Journey* with the results of the search for the reasons for high calcification score, and natural and drug treatment employed to halt the process. It will make a lot more sense to present it to you after we have laid the groundwork for understanding the other risk factors.

## SECOND EBCT SCAN RESULT

The second scan, one year later, calculated a score of 1776, only six points more than the original score of 1770! This was considered an outstanding result and a testament to the regimen of supplements and lipid controls that had been implemented. The calcification had now been stabilized. According to Dr. John Rumberger of the *Mayo Clinic*, a 25-44% increase from the original score of 1770 could have been expected if controls had not been put in place the year earlier. I was not, however, satisfied with the status quo, as I was hoping actually to *regress* the score.

## THIRD EBCT SCAN

I would yet submit to a third scan one year after the second scan to find out how much of the calcification had been reduced. You can imagine my disappointment when **the third EBCT evaluation did not show regression but instead had actually jumped an alarming 910 points to 2,680!** My fibrinogen at this point in time had been brought down and maintained at a safe level over the previous year, so *what* in the regimen had changed and caused this opposite affect? It couldn't have been cholesterol; LDL was in the 70s and the total C was averaging between 150-165.

What had gone wrong between year two and year three? In the meantime I had met Dr. Karol Watson Ph.D, M.D. at *UCLA*, a true advocate of preventive medicine. Dr. Watson knew the area I was exploring intimately, and analyzed the course I had been on to try and determine what could possibly have caused this dramatically in-creased calcification. It was her suggestion to order a second homocysteine test.

*The test confirmed that my homocysteine had risen from 8.7 to 13. Had this increase in (hcy) added the 910 points to the calcification score?*

Nothing else had changed in retesting my previous markers. Dr. McCully's studies had much earlier confirmed rapid atheroslerotic changes had been observed in as short a time as a few weeks in animal studies when high amounts of homocysteine were injected into the mucous membranes of animal subjects. Dr. Malinow's research had proven scientifically that taking niacin caused 50% increased homocysteine levels among test patients. My intake of 750 mgs of niaspan was at least temporarily discontinued and homocysteine levels within a few weeks dropped from 13 to 11 and eventually to 8.3. End of report. Just as CRP guidelines are about to change in 2003, acceptable ranges for homocysteine will most likely be modified in the future. Levels of 13-14 are currently considered acceptable.

# ARTERIOCLEROSIS/ATHEROSCLEROSIS
## (Hardening of the arteries)

As it turns out, the description "hardening of the arteries" used earlier for arteriosclerosis is a very apt one. A surgeon might describe operating on these calcified coronary arteries as similar to cutting through a piece of dry, brittle water hose. While this stage of disease is definitive, I searched to find things that might somehow inhibit the hardening process. Was there nothing to be done to change or ameliorate this status? We know from thousands of studies that antioxidants, which fight free radicals, play a vital role in inhibiting damage to the arterial wall by combating oxidation.

# THE ANTIOXIDANTS

- ▶ E, C
- ▶ coenzyme Q10
- ▶ beta-carotene
- ▶ alpha lipoic acid
- ▶ lutein

- ▶ pycnogenol
- ▶ grape seed extract
- ▶ bilberry
- ▶ zinc
- ▶ turmeric

Garlic and selenium are also among the ammunition that, studies have shown, slow down and neutralize this oxidative form of free radical attack. With my own known amount of calcification already established by EBCT, I would welcome anything that could be added to my regimen that might to any degree slow or possibly even regress the destructive atherosclerosis and arteriosclerosis process. The difference between **arterioslerosis** and **atherosclerosis** is that the source of arteriosclerosis is calcification, while its arterial cousin atherosclerosis uses fatty and oxidative forms of cholesterol byproducts to mount their destruction. A small but illuminating number of studies were done administering the amino acid L-arginine. This amino acid had been proven to offer assistance in maintaining arterial flexibility and suppleness as a strong vosodilator. Nobel Prize winner Linus Paulings led one of these studies, whose findings were released in 1994. Even though Paulings was not a medical doctor, his study had confirmed certain mediating benefits from L-arginine. I therefore began to include 1,500 mgs of daily oral L-arginine in my regimen. *Quite independently*, 7 years after Paulings claims were announced, another Nobel Prize would be awarded to Dr. Louis Ignarro from UCLA and his investigative team for their *most important* breakthrough work on *Nitric Oxide* as a signaling molecule. **L-arginine is a friendly ally, and a natural precursor of nitric oxide.** Defining the clinical pharmacology of L-arginine, Boger and Bode would later publish their findings from the Institute of *Clinical Pharmacology, Medical School, Hannover.*

**Their study proved that arginine is not only a precursor of nitric oxide but also promotes positive endothelium-mediated physiological effects in the vascular system.**

In plain language, this is a good thing! Very importantly, the study further confirmed L-arginine's ability to produce nitric oxide, and therefore **was shown to offer assistance in maintaining suppleness and elasticity in the arteries.** According to the report, several long-term studies have been performed that show:

*" Oral administration of L-arginine or intermittent infusion therapy with L-arginine can improve clinical symptoms of cardiovascular disease in man. "*
—*Boger/Bode*

During this same period of time I had read Linus Paulings' recommendations that some assistance could also be elicited from *L-lysine* (another amino acid), due to its ability to protect vessel and arterial walls. An interesting side note: Paulings was the only individual *ever* to receive *two* Nobel Prizes, and he received them in two very different fields. One award honored his peace initiative, the other his legendary work with cancer and vitamin C. His cardiovascular studies found that certain amounts of *L-lysine* from supplement would compete with and *dissolve arterial plaque* at the artery wall, and that lysine would also have a lowering affect on the inherited gene LP (a). Now we have advice on L-arginine from two recipients of not one but three Nobel Prizes. I was inclined to take their wise counsel, adding 1500 mgs of L-arginine to my regimen with 1500 mgs of L-lysine. Other studies have **identified almonds as a natural source of nitric oxide,** and based on this information, and as an added safeguard, I began including a daily handful of almonds in my diet.

Another statin drug cholesterol study searching for other benefits derived from cholesterol-lowering drug therapy was done at Columbia University. One of the areas of concentration was on *Vasodilation,* a process in which healthy arteries flex inward and outward in response to demands of blood pressure and physical and mental stress. The following favorable results were noted.

1. There had been an increased production of *nitric oxide.*

2. The N/O production improvement proved yet another benefit of statin drug therapy in preserving arterial flexibility. (see *myocardial vasodilation* (MVD).

## LUTEIN AND HEART DISEASE

You might recall having read government health agency recommendations on the importance of consuming five daily helpings of vegetables and fruits, particularly large amounts of the dark green leafy varieties. One of the benefits of this diet would be to assure a proper amount of dietary *lutein* as a weapon against *macula degeneration,* the leading cause of blindness for people entering their senior years. More recently new findings have confirmed additional benefit from fruits and vegetables in *inhibiting oxidation* in the carotid arteries. The article appeared in the *Journal of The American Heart Association* entitled, *A New Vision of Lutein.* A second suggestion from the study was that an increased intake of daily *lutein* may also provide added protection against early **atherosclerosis** as well. The authors based their information on data obtained from representative samples of *diseased carotid artery tissue* removed during surgery. When the tissue was pre-treated with *Lutein* there appeared a marked reduction in the ability of the tissue to attract and involve *monocytes*. This was an important finding because when white blood cells oxidize with LDL cholesterol they destroy artery walls. The authors also reported that the greater the amount of *lutein* supplemented, the lower the amount of *monocyte* interaction. *Here comes another job for the mice!*

---

**The study also confirmed that mice whose diet was supplemented with *lutein* presented a remarkable 43% smaller lesion size than those unlucky mice who had not been given the *lutein*.**

---

**Would this supplement added to my regimen provide added protection? Would it help you? Two months after increasing lutein dosage from 2 mgs to 6,** my blood work showed a 2-point decrease in *monocyte* activity. Looking back at past blood CBC panels over 17 years, this was the lowest the monocytes had ever tested. This record of mono-cyte history might have been an on-going signal of calcification and early endothelium damage. The mono-cytes had always been elevated with the neutrophils on the low side. It turns out there are currently many studies being done on this very association, with an eye on how these two components contribute to the process. I have since increased the lutein intake (3 fold) to 18 mgs. In the final analysis, the only measurement of my overall progress and cardiovascular health would have to be determined from the result of my third thallium treadmill. Dr. Johannes Czercin, M.D., and Director of Nuclear Medicine at *UCLA,* after interpreting the test was convinced that I had the exact cardiovascular results that he would expect to find among his senior athletes. Fortunately, three years later in 2003, the test results remained optimal with a small but increased ejection fraction.

# Chapter 11

# *Crunching* the *Numbers*

## The Grim Statistics from
## The American Heart Association

Research confirms that one person in America suffers a heart attack every 33 seconds, with one death occurring each and every minute. Twenty seven percent of men and **63% of women** experiencing these attacks will expire *within the first year. Fifty percent of all attacks will take the life of their victims within one hour of the first symptom.* The Center for Disease Control in Atlanta calculated the death rate across the board as 40% in 1999. The statistics show that a quarter of a million women will die from heart attacks each year. Among the 1,100,000 initial heart attacks occurring between both sexes in a year, the mortality rate for those patients under the age of 65 will be an alarming 80%.

If this isn't discouraging enough, consider that 48% of these men and 63% of the women had shown NO PRIOR SYMPTOMS before the onset of the attacks. ONE THIRD of those experiencing their first heart attack will die without having a prior warning.

One out of every two eventual deaths in this country will be caused by heart disease in one or more of its various forms. There will be 550,000 new cases of congestive heart failure reported each year with projections of 1.5 million by year 2015. A quarter of a million patients are expected to die in 2003 or in 2004 from sudden death as the result of the illness. **Does one really need to understand the risk factors, and is it incumbent upon you to be involved in your family's cardiovascular health care and diagnostics?** To identify the risk factors long before they manifest themselves in the actual heart attack? Is your family's heart care being treated as a game of *Russian Roulette* with minimal oversight and guidance until a crisis develops? These questions should already have answered themselves. The figures on this illness are overwhelming. The cost, calculated in human tragedy and financial burden, cast upon families and society as a result is staggering per year. All in all, this should make heart disease of paramount concern to all Americans. If we would become a little more knowledgeable, a little more proactive and a good deal more involved with our own healthcare we would be more protective to ourselves and our families.

# Chapter 12

# Stroke Numbers

To the figures reported for myocardial infarction one may add an additional 730,000 of Americans who will be stricken with blood clots and subsequent recurrent strokes in the same year. **Every 53 seconds someone in America will become the victim of a stroke, with one death occurring every 3.3 minutes.** Stroke will claim approximately 159,000 lives in a given year, and therefore ranks as the third largest killer of Americans.

**The *clot* in the vast majority of heart attacks and strokes is the ultimate actual cause of the event. Why then does the clot, and the coagulation and aggregation factors which permit its formation, not receive more demanding risk identification until after the heart attack and after the debilitating stroke have taken their insidious toll?**

Based on knowledge in the past, we believed that if we simply kept our cholesterol at a normal level, say below 200, we would be immune from heart disease. Certainly research has more than suggested that thousands of lives hang in the balance, and that something in the collective thinking and approach needs to be adjusted. The new information does not cancel out what has become known from earlier investigation such as from the Framingham landmark study. The new information you are reading is about the next generation and in most instances a continuation and advancement of the initial study.

# Chapter 13

# *Do* **YOU** *need to become*
# SO INVOLVED?

Consider this: a northern California newspaper, *The Sacramento Bee*, devoted a full page and a half in reprinting an article written by author Michael L. Millenson as previously published in the *Washington Monthly*. The article was entitled DANGEROUS DOCTORS and carried the following subtitle: **"They mean well but they are not keeping up with new research."** The article offered the following advice to its readers:

**"The three words you don't want to say are, 'You're the doctor.' "**
*(sound familiar?)*

This may be so, but could part of the blame be directed at an overtaxed, bureaucratic, micro-managed medical system that places the doctor in a compromised position?

According to Dr. Isadore Rosenfeld, *"You have the right and the obligation to yourself to participate in the decisions that affect your health care."*

## DOCTORS' DEMANDING SCHEDULES

**We, as patients, generally assume automatically that all doctors are aware of all the new information.** There is so much new information for practitioners to absorb that the task becomes almost insurmountable. **It may be years** before a particular doctor becomes aware of certain information and decides to include it in his or her day-to-day practice. This is the information age, and the amount of information for medical professionals to digest is absolutely staggering. Who has the stamina and inclination to look at all that is generated by the information mill? Who has the necessary time? Certainly not any one physician. Not with all the demands a successful practice places on his or her time and energy. Think of all a doctor has to deal with in the course of a given day. Consider also the amount of paperwork needed to comply with agencies and insurance companies no matter how minor the procedure. Consider the constant outpouring of new information a doctor must absorb, not to mention the knowledge they must acquire and maintain related to all the new medications, their implications and side effects. Think of the patient overload, the 30-40 patients to see in a given day plus the coordination and referrals and consultations with specialists—and the need to still have time to visit with their own family and friends. Think of *this* situation (which we seldom hear mentioned). Doctors too, have their own medical problems to contend with after years of stress, overload and the generally poor eating habits necessitated by their work schedules. The practice of medicine is no doubt a daunting one, and yes, they do make a lot of money, but isn't that beside the point?

## THE CRISIS OF THE "TOOs"!

Because of all the factors just listed and more besides, *too* few doctors are seeing *too* many patients, and spending *too* little time with each one. The margin for error and inadequate diagnosis is high. The amount of valuable visitation time is limited. A young dedicated physician, excited about his recent graduation after practicing for a few short months, announced to his family that he would not be continuing in his particular chosen field even though he had devoted many years to becoming a doctor. He explained it this way in recent conversation: *"The way they are teaching us to practice general medicine in the hospital setting is contrary and conflicting to why I became a doctor. I cannot in good conscience rush through my interviews because of the bottom line. Some patients' cases require more time, more investigation, and perhaps more personal attention. Also, because of the many lawsuits leveled at doctors and their associated hospitals, too much of my time is required in looking over my shoulder. I am actually taught to guard what I say, and consequently often times may not be saying enough."* So, after considering what is on the physician's plate, we might want to cut them some slack...but not at the price of accepting anything less than first-class care. You are now becoming more aware as to what constitutes cutting edge analysis and care. In being informed, you will be comfortable that your family is getting the best care available. With all there is available in diagnostics today, the first time one hears that he or she has heart disease should not be when one is lying prostrate on a gurney with the doctor saying ... "Surprise! You have just had a heart attack!" Guess what? Your doctor may be even more surprised than you. That in itself would not be particularly comforting. One thing, however, is becoming abundantly clear and that is: as <u>critical</u> as cholesterol is in the overall equation, *it is not all just a matter of cholesterol!* The other inherited risk factors are becoming recognized and accepted even though mainstream medicine at large does not move quickly to adopt new concepts, regardless of the evidence supporting them. Let's go to school!

*How, then, does one minimize the risks of two of America's leading causes of illness and death? How can you be sure your doctor subscribes to the leading edge diagnostics? How do you alter the odds in your favor for avoiding a debilitating heart attack or stroke? How can you or I know what to ask for or expect with regard to proper identification of our individual risk factors?*

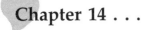

Chapter 14 . . .

# Identifying the "Hidden"
## Heart Attack and Stroke
# Risk Factors

- ▶ *CRP C-reactive protein*
- ▶ *Homocysteine*
- ▶ *Fibrinogen*
- ▶ *ApoB*
- ▶ *Bacterial/viral infections*
- ▶ *Chlamydia pneumonaie*
- ▶ *Helicobacter pylori*
- ▶ *CMV cytomegalovirus*
- ▶ *Herpes simplex*
- ▶ *Lp (a)*

## RISK FACTOR ... # I
### C-Reactive Protein, Inflammation Marker
*Read 'em and Weep!*

C-reactive protein (CRP), is a marker for inflammation and when elevated, a predictor of heart attack and stroke risk, according to Paul M. Ridker, M.D., cardiologist at

*Brigham & Woman's Hospital in Boston MA*, as presented in a report to the **American Heart Association.**

Elevations in CRP have been shown to predict a first heart attack even 6-8 years in advance and were associated with a three time greater risk among men, in the Harvard Physician's Health Study.

## AN INCREASED FIVE-FOLD RISK

High levels of (CRP), the acute-phase reactant protein, marked an increased risk EVEN WITH NORMAL CHO-LESTEROL LEVELS. The risk of future heart attack among those with high levels of CRP AND high cholesterol, according to Dr. Ridker, were greater than the risk of either one individually. High cholesterol by itself could predict a two-fold increased danger, as confirmed in the study.

**However, high cholesterol AND high CRP together WERE ASSOCIATED WITH A FIVE-FOLD INCREASED RISK.**

There have been mountains of health information heaped upon us warning of the risk of cardiovascular disease and the importance of maintaining proper cholesterol levels. How much attention and newsworthy press should be directed at less known inflammatory markers like CRP or fibrinogen? These are factors that individually or in combination can increase one's mortality risk dramatically. Ridker's study reported, in an issue of *Circulation*, that the higher the blood level of CRP, the more likely it is that an older woman will develop cardiovascular disease, *even if she is currently appearing to be in good health.*

## CRP AND A WOMAN'S RISK

(This study has particular significance because it is one of the first CRP studies to include women). The higher the C-reactive protein level among women in the study, the greater the possibility for a heart attack or stroke.

Participants in the highest range of CRP in the study presented a risk **7.3 times higher than other study participants.**

Dr. Ridker, along with his colleagues in ongoing studies, determined that aspirin, as an anti-inflammatory agent, was effective in significantly reducing risk associated with higher than normal levels of C-reactive protein in the blood. **Aspirin therapy used over the eight-year period of the study reduced the heart attack risk by 55.7%.**

Exercise and physical activity have also been shown to lower inflammation levels as was reported in *Epidemiology* 2002;13:561.

**Dr. Oscar O. Bazzino** from the *Italian Hospital* in Buenos Aires, Argentina, as the lead author in a study on CRP, released additional supportive information presented in an issue of *Circulation*. His group's findings also supported the findings of Dr. Ridker's evaluations proclaiming that women with high levels of CRP *had a seven time increased risk of heart attack!* Dr. Bazzino's study concentrated on stable and unstable angina and the CRP connection. Have you or someone you know with heart disease ever been tested for this inflammatory marker? We all should be.

## C-REACTIVE PROTEIN AND ANGINA

The results of a two year study which enrolled 2000 *angina* subjects, published in *Lancet (1997;349:462-6)*, determined that trial subjects whose C-reactive protein levels exceeded 3.6 had a two-fold increase in their individual risk of heart attack or sudden death in comparison with normal subjects. According to the AHA there are 6,400,000 people living with angina in this country alone. The percentage breakdown between men and women affected with angina are very similar. The mounting evidence adds to the speculation that as the body fights to make repairs to damaged vessels, the presence of elevated CRP confounds the results and accelerates a negative outcome. Is it becoming obvious why knowing one's CRP level is vitally important, particularly among heart or stroke patients? There is more.

**Dr. Paul Ridker** and his team's study, *Plasma Concentration of C-reactive Protein and Risk of Developing Peripheral Vascular Disease*, as presented in *Circulation*, vol. 97, issue 5, in 1998, arrived at the following conclusion: *"These prospective data indicate that among apparently healthy men, baseline levels of CRP predict future risk of developing symptomatic **peripheral artery disease** and thus provide further support for the hypothesis that chronic inflammation is important in the pathogenesis of atherothrombosis."* In still another study, which Dr. Ridker and his associates performed at *Brigham and Women's Hospital*, the findings added further support to the theory that, indeed, **heart disease is related to inflammation of the arteries.** The results appeared in the *New England Journal of Medicine*. When 543 physician participants in an 8-year study who had already experienced a heart attack or stroke were compared to the same number of physician participants who had not experienced attacks, the following was learned:

> **Those with elevated CRP levels _but with no evidence of heart disease_ still had three times the risk of suffering a future heart attack and double the risk of having a stroke!**

How would you know if you or a family member had an ongoing inflammatory condition affecting the arterial system and literally threatening your life?

What level of CRP should be considered high? According to the *Physician Study*...

**_THE BASELINE LEVEL_ OF PATIENTS WHO COULD LATER HAVE A HEART ATTACK WAS 1:53 MGS PER LITER; THE NUMBER FOR STROKE VICTIMS WHO COULD EXPERIENCE A STROKE WAS ESTABLISHED AT 1:13.**

Is it not interesting that these 1086 participating subjects were all physicians? Obviously they too are still learning about inflammation's role in heart and stroke disease and, yes, even doctors have heart attacks and strokes.

## SUDDEN CARDIAC DEATH AND CRP

As more and more studies involving this marker are being completed, Dr. Renu Virmani has added another piece to the growing tower of evidence. Dr. Virmani—

associated with and lead investigator of the US Armed Forces Institute of Pathology study in our nation's capital—linked CRP with *sudden cardiac death syndrome,* by analyzing blood samples withdrawn from arteries of 144 women and men who had all died from sudden death. Plaque rupture and/or erosion were proven responsible for 73 of the deaths. The plaques in the remaining 71 were discovered to be stable.

## GUM DISEASE AND CRP

An article appearing in the *Journal of Periodontology* in September 2001 presented the results of a University of Buffalo study whose focus was on how periodontal disease might have a role in the causation of heart disease by elevating CRP levels. The findings proved that patients with the disease recorded the highest concentrations of the marker. Earlier studies had already linked gum and heart disease.

> Could a doctor determine whether or not a patient sitting across the desk from them is positive for HIV or hepatitis C? No, and neither would a doctor know your levels of heart attack risk factors without testing you.

Has the time arrived for adding CRP to annual physical evaluations?

## CRP AND CLAUDICATION

Elevations of CRP, according to study results from the combined efforts of researchers at *Harvard Medical,* are responsible for increased risk of atherosclerosis leading to stroke and heart attack. The study group found that those men with higher levels of CRP had a greater incidence of *claudication* (lower leg pain). Many such individuals, when faced with exertion such as fast walking or running, eventually require surgery for treatment of blocked leg arteries. The diseased arteries have additional difficulty handling the workload because of loss of a significant degree of lumen capacity (open area in the artery) and arterial flexibility. In the study, those men with the highest levels had twice the risk of developing claudication compared to those men whose scores were in the lower ranges. Patients presenting with claudication **need** to be monitored for CRP levels.

Studies have shown that many people without obvious "at-risk profiles for heart disease" have had higher levels of the reactant discovered in their blood streams upon autopsy after their fatal attack.

*C-Reactive Protein* is a marker of current inflammation progression within the body. Other diseases of the inflammatory syndrome can also cause elevations in CRP. Even slight elevations should arouse suspicion, and any elevation above the newest values recommended by Dr. Ridker's investigations must not be dismissed as *normal even though the currently accepted reference charts target much higher numbers as dangerous.* Levels of CRP below 1 mg/l are to be considered low, levels 1-3 are in the moderate range and those levels above 3 according to Dr. Ridker are high. The physician's investigation must then look to the cause. Chapter 16 *The Silent Infections Unmasked* explores many of these suspected microbes. Those patients with any of the following ailments could record higher elevations and would benefit from being tested:

- ▶ Gum Disease
- ▶ Cancer
- ▶ SLE Lupus
- ▶ C. pneumonaie
- ▶ Rheumatoid Arthritis
- ▶ Tuberculosis
- ▶ Heart Disease
- ▶ Pneumonia (Pheumoccocal)
- ▶ Obesity
- ▶ Smoking

The physician may be quick to tell you he or she would expect a higher CRP reading because you have an existing inflammatory condition.

> *While that conclusion would be correct, what is missing from the statement is that the elevation, regardless of the source, has now provided an indirect pathway for the occurrence of a heart attack or stroke.*

The patient wouldn't necessarily die as a direct result of gum disease or any of the other inflammatory illnesses; *it would be the elevated CRP, as a result of the illness, which would cause the heart attack or stroke and possible death of the patient.* This actual cause of the final outcome would probably escape the physician who was not yet aware of the connection between CRP and heart disease. Many physicians use the more familiar ESR test measurement for inflammation, but hi-sensitivity CRP (according to the new research) is a more accurate direct evaluation and the most accurate indicator, especially for evaluating heart and stroke patients' risk. **The current scale for CRP, with 5:0 as the beginning range of high, has and is permitting unnecessary patient risk.**

*Recapping:* according to the *Physician's Health Study,* anything over 1.53 mgs per liter is suspect for possible heart attack and over 1.13 for stroke.

## WOMEN AND CRP

Women with the highest levels of C-reactive protein in the blood (in a study involving 28,000 women), were at much greater risk of having a heart attack or stroke than women in the lower ranges. According to the long- awaited report appearing in the *New England Journal of Medicine,* women recording the highest levels of CRP were 2-3 times more likely to experience a cardiovascular event than those women in the lower ranges. CRP values were shown to be a more accurate predictor of a woman's risk for a heart attack or stroke than even their LDL cholesterol. LDL, which we know as the "bad" cholesterol has until now been considered the most relied upon risk component. The study participants had been monitored over an ongoing 8-year period of time. Insist on a $10-16 (high sensitivity) CRP test.

## SUMMARY

The study of inflammation and inflammatory factors is the *new frontier of cardiovascular research* and application. The collaborative research confirms the vital role of this *acute phase reactant*. At a cost of 10-16 dollars it seems **almost negligent** for anyone not to be tested for CRP during physical examinations. It is a lifesaving test, and certainly as important as the other routine tests regularly performed. The protective, preventive benefit is vital. You might want to request it more specifically as the "cardio" or "hi-sensitivity CRP." Evidence over the past five years of research confirms, if ever there was a marker that cried out for a change in national guidelines it would be C-reactive protein!

### *The Total Evaluation*

Today, before someone can actually know the total risk factors of a particular individual, or be able to point to the specific cause of a given cardiovascular event, the full spectrum of questions must be asked. To simply offer the explanation that the patient has "heart trouble" would be about as vague and useless as your mechanic explaining that your car isn't running because you are having car trouble. "Well, is there a problem with the distributor, transmission, the valves? With our automobiles, don't we want to know, specifically, what is causing the problem? With medicine we plead ignorance; with our automobile we know something about its mechanisms and equipment. We understand much more about the automobile than we do about our own bodies. You are now in the process of changing your base of knowledge.

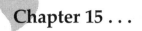Chapter 15 . . .

# *Women*
# *and Heart Disease*

## THE MIS-INFORMATION

It has always been stressed that heart disease is a man's disease and that more men than women die from this ailment. There is in fact a dramatic risk comparison between the two genders.

**For instance, how many people are aware statistically that, during the first year following an initial heart attack, 44% of women will die, compared to 27% of men?**

A British study's findings appeared in the *Journal of the American Medical Association* in October 1998; the abstract was entitled *Women More Likely to Die After First Heart Attack.* How does one make something positive out of this negative information? Might it serve to make women even more aware of their need to proactively safeguard their health?

The study formula was to follow 331 women and 1,129 male patients who had survived a first heart attack. The authors evaluated the subjects 28 days after their attack and again at six months. According to the report, the women presented a 72% greater risk of dying. When the comparison of women's and men's risk evaluation continued, there was a slightly higher 73% risk of a woman dying even six months post heart attack!

## AMERICAN HEART ASSOCIATION'S FINDINGS AFFECTING WOMEN

In 1995, according to the AHA, cardiovascular diseases claimed the lives of more than 505,440 women in the United States. Men's statistics have always gotten the publicity but why have the numbers for women been so downplayed? Men in the same year recorded a lower number of deaths: 455,152. **This amounted to 50,288 more deaths among women in that one year!** What's going on with the information mill? *How many women have been aware of this threat to their health?* We all know the breast cancer and mammogram educators have done a creditable job of making women aware of the breast cancer threat and the need for yearly examinations, but *what about women and heart disease?*

As a woman approaches the age of menopause, her risk increases. It continues to rise with the woman's age. **Men have heart attacks in greater numbers than women—** *however,* **they have them earlier in life.** The difference, according to the AHA, is that *after menopause,* more women do actually die from heart attacks. At this point of their lives women are losing the protective benefit of estrogen.

It is also widely but inaccurately perceived that cancer, (primarily breast and cervical), claims more women's lives than heart disease. As a matter of fact, when asked in survey what is the greatest threat to their health in regard to longevity, women nominate cancer as their first choice. Wrong! Consider the following statistics from the *Department of Health Services.*

**"MORE WOMEN DIE FROM HEART DISEASE THAN FROM ALL MALIGNANCIES** *combined* *including* **BREAST AND CERVICAL CANCER!"**

This is the vital information that has been emerging from health resource databank surveys. Isn't it supposed to just be the man who experiences the chest pain and need for immediate attention? When the same symptoms occur in a woman, they are often explained away as gas or heartburn. Women may recognize the signs of a heart attack in their spouse, but conversely the husband may not recognize the seriousness of the symptoms his own wife is displaying. *"Take some baking soda or antacid and go to sleep."* Because a woman has not been informed about this threat to her own health, she fails, all too often, to understand the symptoms that are signaling the impending or immediate danger. It is even more alarming that (according to various studies), doctors have not been paying enough attention to their female patients' symptoms. **The reason for the lack of concern actually had stemmed from the misconception that heart disease is strictly a man's problem.** A woman may not equate her shoulder, back or chest pain as serious warning signs, and may even hesitate to mention such symptoms to her family, friends or doctor. Most well-meaning people would not think to suggest the possibility of heart disease, preferring a casual diagnostic interpretation of too much tennis, aerobics, golf, floor scrubbing, or nervous tension. You might be amazed to know that heart attacks are occurring even among very young women. Has the medical profession been slow to inform and educate women as to their own risk? A study called the Women's Pooling Project, analyzed the combined results of nine separate studies and concluded that *less than 10% of Caucasian women and less than 5% of African American women would meet the criteria of being "low risk" for heart disease.*

> In other words, 90% of white women were at risk for heart disease while 95% of African-American women were at *significant risk*

## THE GREATER RISK TO BLACK WOMEN

The fact that black women face especially high risk deserves much more conscientious attention.

> The rate of death among black women between the ages of 35-74 is more than 71% higher than the death rate among white women. It doesn't stop there, the death rate comparison overall, between the female counterparts <u>by race</u>, present a higher death rate of 35.3% among black females.

The threat to black women from diabetes is also a major concern. When we see such alarming statistics, one has to wonder if the message is being presented as well as it should be. Look at the stroke equations: **71.4% of black women in the US die from stroke!**

According to Lori Mosca, M.D., Ph.D, Director of Preventive Cardiology at *New York Presbyterian Hospital,* there existed a **3 to 12 fold increased risk of dying of heart disease when those in the higher risk categories were evaluated.** These higher risk categories included obesity, smoking, high blood pressure and or high cholesterol. *Even those individuals with just two risk factors were found to be at increased risk.* Dr. Mosca in her presentation at the *American Heart Association's* annual scientific conference reportedly said: *"despite all that we know about heart disease and its risk factors, the trends in risk factors are worsening."* Our society, remarked Dr. Mosca, is getting fatter; we are doing less exercise, and smoking rates are going down more slowly among women than among men. If this continues, we will face escalating rates of cardiovascular disease. Are not these statistics alarming? In January of 2002, numbers on heart disease and stroke were released: instead of continuing the downward slide that has been occurring during the previous few years, the numbers actually rose. Diabetes (types I & II), which are also vascular diseases, are approaching epidemic proportions. *Obesity,* (over 30 lbs. ideal weight). According to a study in the *American Journal of Clinical Nutrition* an individual's waist size is a greater indicator of heart attack risk than the previously used BMI (body mass index) criteria. The BMI is determined by ones height and weight and has been the standard of measurement for more than 20 years. Nine thousand white men and women took part in the *New York Obesity Research Center* study. The researchers concluded a man enters the danger zone when his waist size reaches 35 inches and a women's risk increased at 33 inches. Other studies have singled out a 40 waist size for men and 35 for women. At these levels, potential of having high cholesterol, higher blood pressure and increased glucose (blood sugar) would be much greater. When these three dysfunctions occur in one profile the condition is called Syndrome X, (see Diabetes and Syndrome X, chapter 29).

## WOMEN, SMOKING AND BIRTH CONTROL

Everyone knows, smoking heightens the risk but *those who smoke and use oral contraceptives* are (according to the AMA) **much more likely** to have a heart attack or stroke.

## WOMEN AND LDL CHOLESTEROL

Dr. Robert Superko, M.D., FACC, and VP of Research of the Berkeley *HeartLab* (associated with the *Lawrence Berkeley National Laboratory),* Berkeley, CA and his investigative team presented the findings of a study at the *American Heart Association's 71st Scientific Sessions.* This particular study had great implications for women's health and inherited risk factors for heart disease. As I mentioned earlier, Dr. Robert Superko and senior scientist Dr. Ronald Krauss are pioneers in the study of genetically inherited heart risk factors. Their work has led to the education of physicians worldwide in identifying other risks as well, including small density LDL particle size and HDL transport particle dysfunction. As complicated as this sounds, it simply means the size of the LDL & HDL cholesterol pieces that are circulating in our blood are of particular importance.

Now for the first time they can be analyzed and controlled.

## LDL PARTICLE SIZE AS ADDED RISK

Superko offered the following explanation and review in his paper entitled *Small Dense LDL: The New Coronary Artery Disease Risk Factor and How it is Changing the Treatment of CAD (coronary artery disease)*. This article was written in 1998 and was revolutionary in its findings.

**"While elevated LDL cholesterol is a risk factor for CAD, the presence of small dense LDL is a more common abnormality, and one that imposes a greater risk than does even elevated LDL."**

The doctor goes on to explain the difference between type "A" patients and type "B" patients. Remember, "A" is the classification we all want and the "B" classification is the one detrimental to our health. According to the report,

*"The small LDL B trait is found in 50% of men with CAD and identifies a group that have a 2 fold greater rate of arteriographic (harmful) progression compared to normal LDL "A" patients."*

Dr. Superko explains that type B individuals have significant success in **favorably altering their status** with the addition of niacin or fibrates and loss of excess weight. In contrast type A people with elevations in their LDL profile do better with *statin* and *resin* therapy as opposed to fibrate therapy. As the information suggests, there is a difference in how a physician might treat individuals who fall into the two different categories. According to the doctor's report, the US health system could save over one billion dollars a year by manipulating these A/B ratio classifications. Blood tests your doctor can order even though this is not normally done will determine which category you are in.

## AN EIGHT-FOLD ADDED RISK
## FOR RECURRENT HEART ATTACKS

A national news health service in discussion with Dr. Arthur Moss from the *University of Rochester* in New York, the lead investigator, presented extremely strong evidence for the relationship between the two blood proteins ApoA1 and ApoB, and a *second heart attack* occurrence. In the study, Dr. Moss's team identified those patients who were presenting elevated levels of the clotting factor D-dimer. The team studied 1000 subjects who had experienced a first heart attack and determined that those individuals who presented with elevated clotting factors and elevated levels of ApoB were *the most destined for a second heart attack*. Moss told the reporter,

**"Individuals who have a tendency to increased blood clotting are at increased risk for recurrent heart attacks, and when you combine this increased clotting with this alteration in the proteins that carry cholesterol, you end up with patients who have an 8 TIMES RISK of recurrent heart attacks, compared with people who don't have these factors."**

We have discussed the difference between ApoA1 and ApoB and how having an elevated ApoB profile (less preferred) produces smaller fat particles that rapidly enter the bloodstream and adhere to arterial walls. It would seem to make sense for anyone with somewhat elevated cholesterol readings or those who have already had a heart attack to know their apolipoprotein status as well as the *dimer* factor. Niacin under a doctor's supervision (along with dietary controls) is the only current therapy to change an individual from an ApoB type to the preferred ApoA. Pursuing this information would require the evaluation of a patient's *D-dimer clotting factor* as well as the apolipoprotein breakdown by a simple blood test and a LDL subfraction electrophoresis study done by a cutting-edge lab, such as The *Berkeley HeartLab*. This is a simple enough diagnostic effort to discuss with your doctor.

## FIBRINOGEN AND LDL PARTICLE SIZE

The 1966 January issue of the *American Heart Association's* journal (ATVB) *Arteriosclerosis, Thrombosis and Vascular Biology* featured a study from Freiburg Germany with Marten Halle, M.D., of the *Medizinische Klinik*. The study concluded *that individuals with elevated fibrinogen levels are indeed at risk for coronary heart disease. Those subjects whose tests results revealed an ability to manufacture the highest number of large, buoyant LDL particles, as opposed to those who produced the much less preferred smaller lighter LDL particles, **were at much less risk with the elevation of their fibrinogen levels.*** A knowledgeable doctor who understands the importance of these sub-fractions may alter and correct these negative factors in your own profile, transforming them to an acceptable scale, *all by natural means.*

## SUMMARY

The side of the breakdown where your blood LDL cholesterol falls can be even more important than high LDL itself. It would be important to know your classification especially since the negative "B" can as a general rule be changed to the preferred "A" class.

Heart disease continues to claim the lives of *half a million* women a year in America. Following a woman's initial heart attack, she remains statistically at significantly greater risk of experiencing a <u>second heart attack</u> within the first year than does a man. Additionally, a woman has a *50% less chance* of surviving the first year of her heart attack compared to the survival statistics awarded her male counterpart. Postmenopausal women beyond age 50, producing decreasing amounts of estrogen are at 3 times greater risk. Women must become involved and proactive in seeking "cutting edge" diagnosis and treatment. To illustrate this need, statistics support the findings that physicians are missing more than one-third of heart attacks even with young patients. A woman's symptoms may be more subtle and must not be dismissed simply because they are not what would be typical in a male. Yes, women need treadmill testing as well as men.

**Risk factors include**: Elevated LDL cholesterol and Triglycerides, low HDL, excessive alcohol consumption, smoking, overweight, hypertension, diabetes, inadequate exercise, stress, and the potential risk of clot formation with high dose birth control medications. *The message:* women need to become informed and proactive in monitoring even subtle symptoms and risk factors.

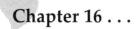

## Chapter 16 . . .

# *Unmasking* the "*Silent*" *Infections*

### CHLAMYDIA PNEUMONIAE ("Cp")
### RISK FACTOR # II, INFLAMMATORY

Not to be confused with the vaginal form of chlamydia, this chlamydia is passed through the air by an airborne respiratory pathogen, not unlike TB or the common cold is transmitted. Opportune infections such as chlamydia pneumoniae (neu-mon-yee), (Cp) may be contracted from someone's cough or sneeze. A simple innocent process in which someone emits thousands of droplets with a single expulsion. This release can propel as many as 30,000 aerosols airborne where they remain suspended for as long as 45 minutes before finally settling. For all intents and purposes this area of air becomes temporarily contaminated. Any person breathing air in this environment is subject to <u>potential</u> infection; consequently, we all have come in contact with this bacterium during our lifetimes. Many of us become actively infected more than once through a process of reinfection because of recurrent exposure to Cp. Four other illnesses under study that are associated with this bacteria are *bronchitis, bronchial asthma, pharyngitis* and *sinutitis*. Chlamydia pneumoniae has now been implicated by a significant number of studies to have an involvement with the development of heart disease. One study reported in the journal *Circulation*, led by Dr. Michael Davidson, from *Johns Hopkins University School of Hygiene and Public Health*...

> *It was learned that when the arteries of deceased subjects were confirmed to have high levels of Cp., they proved to be* **TEN TIMES** *more likely to have the bacteria found in coronary lesions.*

When these results were compared to those who had been diagnosed with either a minor degree or no infection at all, it was determined that these subjects may have previously **become infected as long as 5 to 14 years before their death.** Presence of this bacterium is particularly harmful to cardiovascular health when the infection (albeit a low-grade one) has remained unidentified and dormant in our systems for many years. Cp in its contagious stage produces flu-like systems which may include fever, malaise, dry hacking cough, wheezing, and chill, possibly accompanied by soreness in the chest as an obvious result of continued coughing. Cross infection may occur, developing into other respiratory ailments and involve the commonly recognized *mycoplasma pneumonia, H. pylori, (CMV) cytomegalovirus)* and possibly herpes simplex. **Here again it would seem prudent to be tested, particularly if one has presented with other risk factors or indications of heart disease or if one has already experienced a heart attack.** Cp became suspect when it was first found in atherosclerotic tissues and plaques. A study in 1988, appearing in the European journal *Lancet,* linked coronary heart disease to Cp when the study results **found that subjects with low-grade infection were more likely to develop heart disease than those with healthier profiles.** There have been numerous studies that have confirmed finding Cp bacteria present in plaques.

When C. pneumoniae was injected into the bloodstreams of animal subjects (namely rabbits and mice) **these animals quickly developed arteriosclerosis in the aorta (the body's main artery). This acute respiratory pathogen is associated specifically with heart attack, arterial, carotid and cerebrovascular (brain) disease.**

## IS CORONARY HEART DISEASE
## AN INFECTIOUS DISEASE?

The research concentrated on the possible role of C. pneumoniae and heart attack in patients under age 65 in an issue of the journal *Chest* in August of 97. The investigative team at the *University of Milan* was under the leadership of Dr. Francesco Blasi. The study involved 61 patients who had endured a myocardial infarction. In the study's testing it was learned that *23 of the 61 had chronic or lingering Cp infection.* Twelve patients showed that they had become re-infected from earlier exposure to Cp. Of the total 61 subjects, **35 tested positive.**

> What is surprising is the fact that these twelve patients (almost 20% of the group) had suffered a recent respiratory tract infection <u>within the three-week period before having their heart attacks</u>.

## ANTIBODIES

While anyone who has acquired this disease in their lifetime will have developed antibodies, it remains very difficult for even a knowledgeable physician to determine if these antibodies are presently active. The common tests are the IgG and IgM antibody tests. The conclusions of the *West Birmingham Stroke Project* appearing in the journal *Stroke*, Vol. 29 1998, found an association between stroke and C. pneumoniae as reported in their abstract entitled *Chlamydia pneumoniae antibody titers are significantly associated with acute stroke and transient cerebral ischemia*.

## ANTIBIOTICS CAN ELIMINATE Cp

*When antibiotics that had been proven effective in controlling chlamydia were taken within the prior 3 years, fewer overall heart attacks were recorded.*

One thing for sure; patients won't be able to determine they are destined for a heart attack in the approaching three years, and will never know if they are positive for Cp, unless doctors begin testing their heart disease patients. Particularly if an elevation in the infection marker (CRP) is noted. Studies conducted at *John Hopkins* and *Louisiana State University* found that indeed this pathogen did affect the cells that are involved with the actual construction of atherosclerotic lesions or plaques, and from the findings determined that this respiratory pathogen <u>does</u> play a role in the causation of heart attacks.

> **Researchers learned, in still more studies performed in other countries, that when chlamydia pneumoniae was injected into the mucous membrane of the noses of rabbits, most of them *developed plaques in their arteries* within just seven weeks!**

I have chosen to include these many different studies in supporting Cp's involvement with heart disease simply because the medical community has at this point not ruled definitively on it's involvement. There appears to be enough evidence to indicate a need, at least from a preventive standpoint, for patient testing and elimination of this bacterium. The enclosed information you are being presented may be helpful in your discussion with your physician. Studies have shown that the drug azithromycin (Zithromax) has been the most effective in treating C. pneumoniae. Another antibiotic named *roxithromycin* in the beginning of 2003 has offered hope as another weapon in the treatment of Cp. *Tetracycline* has been shown to be a much less effective alternative. Wouldn't it be prudent for patients diagnosed with heart disease to ask their doctors about including this blood test?

## SUCCESS IN ELIMINATING INFECTIONS

A study on antibiotic treatment for both H. pylori and C. pneumonaie divided its enrollment into two separate groups. One would receive antibiotic therapy, and the other would receive none. The results at the end of six month's therapy were as follows: Subjects in the treated group who had been designated positive at the outset of the study for helocobacter pylori (H.pylori) had eradicated the infection entirely from their systems in 35 of the 37 cases. The testing results among the subjects who had been identified positive for C. pneumoniae at the outset indicated a significantly decreased presence of C. pneumoniae. As a result of treatment there was also a very significant decrease in the patient's fibrinogen levels (an important inflammatory independent risk factor) in both groups of patients involved with antibiotic therapy. Those volunteers monitored in the control group (who did not receive antibiotic therapy) actually *increased their fibrinogen levels* by 45 points. As study has continued on these inflammatory agents, additional results suggest that even more viral and bacterial infections may be connected with heart disease. Another example is offered by Dr. David Siscovick, a professor at the University of Washington, exploring whether or not inflammation played a causative or related role in heart disease. Two hundred of the 600 subjects; *had already experienced a previous myocardial event*. Not only did the study concentrate on Cp, but also evaluated two other infections: *herpes simplex* and *cytomegalovirus* (CMV). According to the published results, *those individuals who have been infected with the herpes simplex type 1 virus (categorized as **HSV-1**) are more likely to have a heart attack than those who have not been exposed to it.* You cannot eliminate an infection that your doctor doesn't know you have.

> **This herpes classification often expresses itself physically in cold sores. The research implies that those who have been infected have twice the propensity for experiencing, or even dying from, heart disease compared to those who have not been infected.**

This obviously doesn't mean that anyone who has had a cold sore or genital herpes is going to die of heart disease! Note: *cytomgalovirus* and *Epstein-Barr* are also of the herpes family and under suspicion as contributors to this phenomenon. A total of eight microbes including the bacterial infection *Hemophilus* influenzae associated with ear and upper respiratory infections are also on the study agenda. At this date the jury remains out.

## HOW LONG HAS Cp BEEN SUSPECT IN HEART DISEASE?

As early as I could ascertain, the pathogen came under the microscope for its involvement in heart disease in 1988 as recorded in *Lancet* by a Dr. Saikku. The study showed, possibly for the very first time, a correlation between this bacterium and *myocardial infarction (MI)*. A subsequent study appeared in *Annals of Internal Medicine* and focused on information derived from the landmark *Helsinki Heart Study*. In short, the germ has been under suspicion for a fairly long time.

## SUMMARY

Even though the puzzle is now much more complete, there are physicians who *still* question the role Cp, and other infections play in heart disease and whether or not drug therapy provides an effective and necessary treatment. **The preceding information presented should serve to dissuade much of that doubt.** If you have had repeated episodes of upper respiratory illness or bronchial asthma, you might want to discuss having this test performed with your doctor.

# Chapter 17

# Homocysteine

## Risk Factor # III

We have briefly touched on *homocyst(e)ine*, (hcy), a sulfur-containing amino acid involved in *methionine* metabolism as a product of *methionine*. Homocysteine (homo-cys-teine) has now finally been recognized as an independent risk factor for heart disease and stroke. L-cysteine, another of the amino acid family, is involved in rendering homocysteine harmless as it assumes a pivotal role in a conversion process known as *remethylation*. In this process (hcy) is transformed into a harmless state. *Homocysteine* was a new word added to the public's vocabulary as it began appearing for the public's consumption in magazine articles and various TV commercials promoting the sale of products to protect the system against inadequate amounts of *folic acid*. Some might have even wondered upon first hearing if this new word was a politically correct one! Homocysteine's link to heart disease was first recognized more than 30 years ago by a young pathologist named Kilmer McCully. To be duly accurate, there had been an earlier *flirting* notion of an involvement in a case of homocyst(e)inema (ho-mo-cys-tein-enima) by a physician in Ireland in the early sixties. Homocysteine is also involved in an adverse platelet aggregation process which can begin a cascade of events eventually leading to fatal heart attacks and strokes. Homocysteine has been shown to be *strongly involved* with the oxidation of "bad" (LDL) cholesterol. Levels of hcy which are currently accepted as normal should in fact (as you will see) be rejected in favor of lower levels. It is a fact that homocysteine negatively influences heart disease in general, and especially carotid and peripheral disease.

## HOW HIGH IS HIGH?

Several recent studies have differed in their findings from what the medical profession has considered acceptable. One meta-analysis study presented at an International Stroke Conference in 2000 focused on mild-to-moderate (hcy) elevations and stroke. The meta-analysis study of 35 individual studies led by Peter J Kelly identified a dramatic **86% increased** stroke risk **in even *mildly* elevated cases.** This adverse complication, interestingly, was found *in the absence* of, and independently of, what would normally qualify as <u>high</u> LDL or triglyceride levels. In conclusion: consider the collective evidence.

> **There is a much greater risk for both stroke and heart disease than we have been led to believe by what the medical profession has determined to be "normal" levels.**

For those patients diagnosed with SLE (Lupus) disease, stroke risk is magnified and homocysteine levels should become an even greater concern. Elevated levels have been identified as causing hardening and thickening of the walls of the carotid arteries. To answer the questions "how high is high" and what level you as a patient should accept in your own healthcare, we look to the 1995 journal *Circulation's* November 15 issue. The article had reported that **values above 6.3 produced a rapid escalation of heart attack risk**. Other studies have narrowed the ideal safe range between 6.3 and the number 7. Standard charts being used by labs across the country show 15 as the threshold of the danger zone. We know we can't always rely entirely on what we read. Just last year the cholesterol ranges that have been adhered to as gospel for more than fifty years were finally amended. A new medication that is touted as the greatest life saving drug for a particular disease within a year is proven responsible for the deaths of 15 patients and removed from the shelves. There is little doubt among researchers that homocysteine safe values on charts will be re-evaluated. Common sense, aligned with scientific scholarship, will dictate the change. As a designated "independent risk factor," this amino acid lines up with such other risk factors as smoking, high cholesterol and high blood pressure. Expensive pharmaceutical drugs are not the answer here. Perhaps that has been part of the problem; it might help explain why homocysteine has had relatively minor attention as a cardiovascular risk factor until recently. The normal therapy for managing homocysteine is a combination of the B amino (folic acid), taken with B6 and B12. B12 also offers added protection against a rare but serious ailment, *pernicious anemia*. It is amazing that a remedy costing only a few pennies a day could affect the life and death of an individual. For the most part the received wisdom has been that an individual taking 400-420 mcgs of folic acid, (micrograms as opposed to milligrams) should be provided sufficient prophylaxis. However, this standard amount does not always provide the necessary protection, as several studies have shown. Patients whose levels, if tested, would have proven to require a much larger dosage than the standardized recommended 400-420 mcgs of folic acid. *Dr. Rene Malinow* of the *Oregon Health Sciences Center* in Portland is one of the most knowledgeable scientists studying homocysteine. He has devoted many years to investigating and monitoring the risks associated with elevations of this amino acid. *He believes certain individuals may actually inherit this dysfunction.* To give you an idea of how important it is to control escalating homocysteine levels, Dr. Malinow has said *"Increasing folic acid levels would immediately prevent 50,000 deaths from vascular causes each year."* Sixteen medical centers of the *European Concerted Action Project* studying homocysteine reported that among 750 study subjects taking supplements to inhibit homocysteine, a significant number of patients presented with two thirds less risk of vascular events. Beginning in 1984, studies originating in the Netherlands, Japan and New York supported the basic conclusion that higher homocysteine levels are found among subjects with heart disease when compared to those with lower levels. Other research has linked hcy with all of the various processes that result in arteriosclerotic plaque development. The theory is that damagingly high toxic levels deposited in blood vessels invite an inverse relationship with LDL cholesterol and, consequent formation of *plaque*. Testing, particularly among patients who have a family history of stroke or heart disease or for those who continue to smoke, would make sense. This however is not the current standard approach.

## THE GOOD NEWS

As a matter of fact, whether or not you have the test the treatment would, *under normal situations*, be the same: 420 mcgs of folic acid along with 100-200 mgs of B6 and 800 mgs of B12. Both folic acid and B12 are reported to be generally well tolerated, however, B6 dosage above 100 mgs can become toxic. With those with homocysteine levels in the highest ranges, a doctor (respecting the new findings) would probably more readily achieve success by adding not only more folic acid but also two other supplements to establish the proper threshold. *Increasing folic acid alone would probably not bring about the desired result.* In controlling higher levels of homocysteine, the addition to the regimen of N-acetylcysteine (l-cysteine) has been proven to reduce high homocysteine by 45%. Betaine in its natural form of Tri-Methyl Glycine (TMG) is particularly effective when used in combination with B6, B12 and folic.

## TO TEST OR NOT TO TEST?

Here, however, lies a potentially serious problem. Most doctors would not choose to administer a homocysteine test at a cost of approximately $145-175. The doctor might explain this to the patient and the service provider by saying that the intake of 400 or 420 micrograms of folic acid is all that is necessary for adequate protection. Many doctors may suggest that taking that amount daily would remove the need for the additional cost of a test. *This argument is almost right*, but may be penny-wise and pound-foolish. There is a new test available that should make the insurance company a lot happier: it costs only $80! Ask your doctor for the *Abbott* Homocysteine Test.

**The patient might find, by taking the test, that he or she requires much higher amounts of folic acid than 420 or even 800 mcgs to remedy and neutralize high homocysteine.**

The patient and the physician, without testing, could only guess if this were the case, and might extend the patient's risk without even being aware of it. Based on the evidence, elevated homocysteine is a serious concern and it would seem to be almost irresponsible to not be tested.

## HEAVY COFFEE AND MEAT CONSUMERS RAISE THEIR HOMOCYSTEINE

Those patients indulging in heavy meat high protein diets are at risk of elevated  homocysteine levels.  The Atkins diet is back in style, if you try it you might consider monitoring your  homocysteine. Dr. Atkins is a cardiologist who advocates a very effective high protein, meat and low carb diet. Coffee drinkers consuming more than **2.5 cups of coffee per day** might be raising their homocysteine levels. It is certainly not difficult to extrapolate from the study that if as little as 2.5 cups have been shown to raise homocysteine levels, then those coffee drinkers who have one or two cups in the morning and another two at lunch or dinner, on top of what they drink during the day at work, may be according to the information, raising their levels significantly. We are, as the corner coffee shops would indicate smack dab in the coffee generation. Those who drink large amounts of coffee might require additional folate and supplements to attain and maintain compliance. A study out of Oslo Norway published in the August 2001 issue of the *American Journal of Clinical Nutrition* showed a 10% *decrease* in homocysteine levels among study participants who abstained from drinking coffee over a six-week period. Another study found that **decaffeinated coffee did not cause an increase in (hcy) levels**. It has been pretty well accepted through the years that heavy coffee drinkers expel great amounts of B vitamins in general. This new information is more specific, and addresses folic acid in particular. A Dr. Charalambos Vlachopoulos reporting on his study from the *Cardiology Department of the Henry Duanat Hospital* of Athens, Greece, found that the arteries actually temporarily "hardened" and remained hardened for several hours after drinking *a single* cup of coffee. While we are on this subject of *passive* causes of arterial hardening, an article from the Australian Baker Medical Research Institute, under the leadership of Dr. Paul Nestel, found that study subjects given a high fat meal consisting of 50 grams of fat (in the form of a ham and cheese sandwich accompanied by a glass of whole milk and followed by ice cream as dessert) showed a reduction of up to a 27% overall elasticity in the large arteries. There are also other factors involved in passive and permanent "hardening of the arteries."

## VISP (VITAMIN INTERVENTION FOR STROKE PREVENTION TRIAL)

"The truth shall set us free" trial was designed to determine what amounts of B6, B12, and folic acid are actually required to minimize the risk of additional strokes to those who have already experienced one or more strokes.

This trial is on-going and promises to be a significant advance in the area of stroke. The study is sponsored by the NIH (National Institute of Health). It would serve to further support the notion that one universal amount of 400 mcgs of folic acid is most certainly not therapy enough to settle all cases. The folic acid dosage used in the study is 2500 mcgs. A major study like this might take 20 years.

## HOMOCYSTEINE AND OTHER DISEASES?

At this time, homocysteine has been implicated in the causation of heart disease, stroke, Alzheimers, general dementia, neural tube fetal spinal development in infants and is currently being studied as a possible factor in other ailments including colon cancer. Researchers from **Harvard University released study data confirming that of 88,000 women in their study, those with familial history of colon cancer were able to reduce their risk by 50% with folic acid supplements!** Other women in the study without family history of this form of cancer found a 19% risk reduction from taking folate. This according to the information released in the publication *Cancer, Epidemiology, Biomarkers and Prevention* in an August 2002 edition. The following information appearing in the *European Journal of Clinical Investigation* confirms homocysteine's role in increasing the debilitating incidence of stroke.

*40% more embolic and hemorrhagic strokes occurred among those stroke victims with elevated homocysteine levels.*

These are significant numbers, and patients might want to demand closer preventive monitoring of their levels. At the risk of redundancy, most physicians and general laboratories rate a level of 14-15 as a point of concern. As you read the following study, you will be able to draw your own conclusions as to what you should accept as low, middle or high in your own profile.

## "A SILENT STROKE EPIDEMIC"

Four papers were presented at the *American Stroke Association* and together they revealed the alarming role homocysteine is playing in the number of "silent" strokes. Most of us associate a stroke with either immediate death or paralysis of part of the anatomy, such as the face, legs or perhaps an arm. Here, the results of the stroke are physically manifested and are obvious to the observer. However, as the researchers at the conference revealed, there is a newly discovered phenomenon, and homocysteine appears to be in part at the very root of it. According to the research, these *silent strokes* do not take an obvious immediate toll, but rather do their insidious damage cumulatively over years. We recognize that stroke damage becomes obvious when it affects the speech, the walk, the facial countenance and certainly one's ability to think, to move and to remember. This newly identified form of stroke does not necessarily cause the traditional signs of damage that physicians are accustomed to identifying. These strokes may have been happening to a patient for years unrecognized by doctors or even the victim. There is more.

## MILDLY ELEVATED HOMOCYSTEINE
## LINKED TO 11 MILLION STROKES PER YEAR

According to the findings, **11 million people are experiencing silent strokes annually in addition to the 750,000** who have experienced strokes with all the classic identifiable results. While the medical profession is just beginning to become accustomed to the idea that high levels of homocysteine might be dangerous, the truth appears to be that even "mildly" elevated levels are damaging. This new information prompted Dr. Magen C. Leary, from UCLA, to say:

*"* **Silent Strokes Are Epidemic In This Country.** *"*

These strokes (according to Dr. Leary) do not inflict visible damage because they occur in parts of the brain where the symptoms are not immediately recognized. Dr. Leary has suggested, "The word 'silent' be put in quotes, because the effects accumulate over the years." Apparently the cumulative damage over time shows up in a patient's memory loss, mood changes and difficulty with mobility. All are signs that we commonly accept as products of old age. Dr. Leary drew her conclusions regarding "silent" brain attacks after studying some 5,500 brain scans. What is of particular significance is how many other recent research papers are supporting the same basic findings. A study that looked at high homocysteine and dementia (as reported by F. Lebihuber and team in *Journal of Neural Transmission* (issue 12, 2001) found significantly elevated hcy levels among both patients with *vascular dementia* and Alzheimer's disease. The report claimed a significant correlation between *low* folic acid concentrations and cognitive decline. In a report entitled *"Early Diagnosis of cognitive in the elderly with focus on Alzheimer's disease,"* C. G. Gottfries and B. Regland found homocysteine levels to be an early and sensitive marker for cognitive impairment. There are numerous studies that prove a link between homocysteine levels and "short term memory" loss. A Tufts University study found that patients with higher hcy scores were 30% less efficient on memory tests compared to those who had lower levels. In May 2001 the *American Journal of Clinical Nutrition* carried the favorable results of a study in which participants who had taken higher amounts of folic acid showed a greater ability to recall the details of a story.

## THE NEGATIVE 50% + ASSOCIATION BETWEEN NIACIN AND HOMOCYSTEINE

Niacin (which is being prescribed more than ever before for its role in maintaining proper cholesterol profiles) can have a devastating influence on homocysteine. An article appearing in the *Journal of the American Heart Association* 1999; 138:1082-7 was entitled, *Niacin treatment increases plasma homocyst(e)ine levels.* According to the study by Dr. Malinow and the *ADMIT* investigative team, niacin can actually **increase homocysteine levels as much as 50%!** Since the release of findings concerning meeting and maintaining optimum cholesterol levels, niacin has been used successfully to raise HDL and lower LDL, and for total cholesterol management. It is also a component of combination therapy in difficult cholesterol profiles. It has been prescribed more in the past five years because of the new concerns raised by researchers concerning low HDL as an important risk factor. It very often is prescribed in the form of *niaspan* for its positive role in converting a patient's *subfraction* profile from an undesirable type B to type A. It has also been credited with controlling HDL transport conversions as well as mediating against an inverse LP (a) dysfunction. It is a *wonder drug* and from all indications should be treated as a drug, particularly when taken in large amounts, even though 1500 mgs have been generally well tolerated. Dr. Rene Malinow, Rekha Garg and their team proved niacin's unholy alliance with homocysteine. The benefits of niacin therapy for many patients are clear and significant and throwing the *baby out with the bath water* would not be the wise suggestion. The prudent approach here would seem to be to adjust the amount of folic acid and other control supplements taken in accordance with the test results.

## THE HOMOCYSTEINE BEGINNING

Here is another frustrating example of how long it can take for vital information to migrate from the research community to final acceptance in mainstream practice. Homocyst(e)ine was found to be a possible link to heart disease more than 30 years ago by a young professor of pathology at Harvard Medical School named Kilmer McCully. McCully in the 70's proffered the theory, based on his research, that a rarely identified genetic dysfunction called *homocystinuria* had been the direct cause of premature arteriosclerosis in three earlier cases involving very young subjects.

> The third case history, according to McCully, revealed startling information: that a two-month-old subject at the time of his death had already presented with *homocystinuria* and consequent advanced arteriosclerosis.

Dr. McCully began supporting his belief with animal studies, and found an independent study which had been performed in Seattle Washington had shown dramatically, that when homocysteine was infused in primates *arteriosclerotic plaque* was readily produced. The pathologist in his own study produced similar results when infusing homocysteine into the noses of rabbits. The dye had been cast. He therefore now hypothesized, based on his findings and supporting evidence, that elevated homocysteine would do the same in humans. The theory was met with great disdain, (according to the pathologist) it even became a source of humor. It apparently must have been unthinkable at the time to speculate that this seemingly inconsequential substance produced by the body could be the origin of such serious consequences as "hardening of the arteries" and actual heart attack and stroke. At the time, the theory appeared to be ridiculous on its face. After all, medical science was at that time just beginning to come to grips with the notion that something called cholesterol was the cause of heart disease. McCully's theory was woefully out of step with the establishment. When he made his presentation and produced his results (as he would later explain), students and colleagues were rudely talking among themselves, and some actually walked out during his presentation.

## REDEMPTION

Call it poetic justice, but almost 26 years after McCully's untimely departure from the university, this same medical school enlisted 271 men for a study on guess what? Homocysteine. The study confirmed many of McCully's earlier findings, garnering support for his earlier claims. The Harvard study was a very important one in moving the homocysteine factor forward as they have been on the cutting edge of cardiovascular research. The study concluded that men with high levels of homocysteine in their blood were in fact putting themselves at **a three or four times higher risk of heart attack** when compared to those in the lower ranges of the comparison scale. Actually it is not unusual for the discoverer of a medical breakthrough to meet with strong resistance. This sadly seems to have been the case with most research breakthroughs. After all, didn't it take some forty years before the stethoscope was readily and generally accepted? Was not the great Lister himself denied respect for his claim that something called germs or bacteria were unconsciously being carried into the operatory on the hands and clothes of doctors dissecting and studying cadavers? These germs, although not visible to the naked eye, were actually causing the deaths of thousands of people? Ridiculous! Outrageous! Germs, why how important could they be, you can't even see them!

## HOW IT WORKS

As a general rule the body controls homocysteine because it has the ability to convert it to a non-toxic compound called cystathionine. The problem surfaces when the body is deficient in vitamin B6 and folic acid. One has to admire Dr. Julian Whitaker for the unsolicited apology he made several years ago for the entire profession when he wrote:

**"It was right there in front of us all the time and we didn't see it. I must now apologize to my patients and tell them homocysteine may be the death of half of us."**

Are you among those currently at risk? With all due respect, without being tested, how would you know if the 400 micrograms of folic acid that has suddenly been added to your daily vitamin bottle or favorite cereal is sufficient to meet the specific amount your body requires? Dr. Malinow, from the *Oregon Health Center*, whose work has been published in peer journals more than 50 times on this particular subject, believes certain individuals *do inherit a genetic dysfunction in homocysteine synthesis.* How would these patients fare seeking protection from only the minimum amount of folic acid? In fact it was his article in the journal of the *American Heart Association* that made me realize that distinct elevations in my homocysteine might well have been caused directly by an increased intake of **Niacin.** Cessation of niacin for three weeks produced a marked almost 5 point reduction in my (hcy) level. As McCully has come to be considered an excellent pathologist, other members of the profession, researchers, scientists and physicians, have joined the battle and hoisted their banners. These individuals have dedicated much of their careers to examining this homocysteine phenomenon, performing additional in-depth studies and trials to further confirm, or deny, the homocysteine threat: *Drs H. Mudd, M.J. Stampfer, R. Rozen, and J. Finkelstein,* to name a few. Collectively they have continued to suggest still more benefits from maintaining proper homocysteine levels. These professionals and many others (some of whose work is included in this book) are involved in on-going trials and studies which have concentrated on homocysteine's role in contributing not only to the ravages of heart disease and stroke, but to other diseases as well. With an aging population, dementia and Alzheimer's are a major health concern, and early indications point to elevated homocysteine's possible role in these ailments. There is an interesting addition to this discussion of dementia. A study completed at the *National Institute of Aging*, Bethesda, Maryland, confirmed a **300% increased risk for all dementias combined, including Alzheimers** among the participants with the higher levels of the (inflammatory marker, C-reactive protein). Study author Lenore J. Launer reported in the *Annals of Neurol* 2002;52. We have been reading about two possible risk factors, (*homocysteine* and *C-reactive protein*), that suggest inflammation as a potential route for the increase in dementia and Alzheimers disease in America. More studies are currently in progress.

## ALZHEIMERS/HOMOCYSTEINE LINK

Homocysteine has been one of the subjects of more than 150 studies including the *Framingham, the Physician Health Study and the European Tromso Study*. A new study or article on homocysteine appears in journals every day, and many of the new studies are aimed specifically at determining links between (hcy) dementia and Alzheimers. The general consensus of no less than fifty studies is that homocysteine levels are linked to both illnesses. One study determined that test patients with Alzheimer's disease presented an elevated homocysteine score when compared to non-Alzheimer patients in the same study. These study findings were announced by British researcher Dr. David A. Smith of the *University of Oxford*, in the UK, who presented the study findings at the *American Medical Association's (AMA) conference* in Durham, North Carolina. Dr. Smith and his team divided the study subjects into two classifications: 164 patients who had previously been diagnosed with Alzheimer's disease, and 108 study subjects of the same ages (over 55) without the disease. The following findings were the result:

> **Those with the *highest* level of homocysteine were FOUR AND A HALF TIMES MORE LIKELY TO DEVELOP ALZHEIMER'S DISEASE.**

This was the determination when the *higher* study scores were compared to those patients with the *lowest* level. Dr. Smith proclaimed an urgent need for further studies. Here again a study provides a possible link between folic acid levels and Alzheimer's disease. *Total Serum Homocysteine in Senile Dementia of Alzheimer Type* is the title of a study by McCaddon and team that appeared in the *International Journal of Geriatric Psychiatry*. Among the conclusions drawn from the study was support for the idea that minor deficiencies of B12 occur more frequently among senile dementia patients than among healthier elderly patients, and are initially indicated by higher homocysteine levels.

## A LARGE STUDY WITH ASTOUNDING IMPLICATIONS

Dr. Jeremy D. Kark of Hadassah University Hospital, Jerusalem, Israel and his team at two separate sites, Israel and Boston MA's Tufts University, as reported in the *Annals of Internal Medicine*, found that even *when "mildly" elevated levels of homocysteine are present there is an increased risk of death from any cause.* The study enrolled some 1,788 subjects. Dr. Kark reported that those patients whom he described as having MILDLY elevated homocysteine levels had a 30%-50% higher risk of death than those with the lowest levels. The researchers came to these findings over a 9-11 year study, concluding that the actual risk of death was **twice as high** among people with the highest levels of homocysteine when compared with those re-cording the lowest levels. As alarming as what you have just read about homocysteine, the information you will be presented on fibrinogen will prove similarly as dramatic. There are more than 185 studies that have basically con-firmed homocysteine's role in heart disease. *The Physician's Health Study* claimed that the risk was over three times higher among subjects in the top 5% of those tested in their study. This condition, called *hyperhomocysteinemia*, was found in another study in 20-30% of CAD patients. *Could the reason it is found among CAD patients be be-cause* **it was the actual reason they became CAD patients in the first place?**

## "HARDENING OF THE ARTERIES"

In the past this term "hardening of the arteries," was commonly employed to describe the process that is more formerly known as heart disease or arteriosclerosis. Studies have identified (hcy) in components of both arterial and venous disease where it attacks the endothelium. It is here where homocysteine is believed to cause negative *thrombalytic* response, dangerously increasing LDL oxidation. Here is yet another example of why antioxidants are important and why trans and saturated fats must be avoided with disdain. As this information is being compiled, much research at the pharmaceutical level is being aimed at developing medica-tions to interfere with the process of LDL oxidation. In this process, the LDL cholesterol becomes oxidized, entering — and damaging—the vessel wall as free radicals. Trans fats, of course, also hasten this process, and recent studies have proven trans fats are even more destructive than saturated fats. Many people who indiscriminately ingest an excessive amount of beta-carotene may also unknowingly be augmenting their risk. The endothelium lining and the arteries themselves normally enjoy an ability to constrict or enlarge (dilate) in a rubber-band-like fashion in order to quickly meet increased blood flow demands placed upon the body. These demands are made in response, for example, to physical exertion or mental stress. When arteries lose their elasticity or flexibility they are unable to respond adequately to meet the demands. A heart attack or stroke too often is the result.

## HOMOCYSTEINE & CANCER?

Additional research suggests another possible cancer link, namely that low levels of folate in the body predispose one to damaging their DNA, a process that encourages cancer cells to proliferate. Now that you have the benefit of these and other prominent studies you can discover *this* hidden heart attack and stroke facilitator in time to protect yourself. That is the good news. Dr. Rachael Stolzenberg-Solomon of the National Cancer Institute in Bethesda, Maryland **reported on a link between _pancreatic cancer_ (one of the most deadly forms of cancer) and smoking.** It appeared in a 4/2001 issue of the *American Journal of Epidemiology*. Briefly, of the 27,000 men who were followed in the study, 157 developed pancreatic cancer. The researchers supported the earlier findings of the *American Cancer Society*, which had determined that smoking and a high fat diet significantly raised the risk of this fifth deadliest form of cancer.

Those men in the study who ate the richest folate (folic acid) diet exhibited one half the risk of developing cancer when compared to those men who ate the least. Folate, according to the study, offered some protection against pancreatic cancer among those who smoked.

The point here is that cancer is yet another disease where folate may be offering some protection in one's overall risk profile.

## SAME AS SMOKING A PACK A DAY

This study should be of particular interest to smokers. According to the report, the amount of damage from elevated homocysteine may equate to having smoked one pack of cigarettes a day over the same time period! Not good! That is what a professor from the *University of Maryland School of Medicine,* has claimed. According to Dr. Steven J. Kittner, a neurology, epidemiology and preventive medicine doctor writing in a journal *Stroke* report, "The magnitude of the increase in stroke risk was similar to that of smoking a pack of cigarettes a day."

*"Even moderately higher homocysteine levels—as those that would be considered normal in older people—conferred a greater risk of stroke among women in our study."*

# HIGH HOMOCYSTEINE LEVELS
# IMPLICATED IN WOMEN'S STROKE RISK

Now, even women's stroke risk seems to implicate homocysteine as a contributor. Those with high levels have *twice the* risk of those with normal levels. Researchers from the *University of Maryland* studied homocysteine levels in some 167 women ages 15-44. Each of the study subjects enrolled in the program had already experienced a stroke. The study looked at a group of 328 women who had not had a stroke. When traditional risk factors such as smoking and domestic pressures were included, *those women with the highest levels of homocysteine were still 60% more at risk for an episode with stroke* than the women with the lowest levels. Levels of homocysteine among post-menopausal women frequently rise matching levels found in men. As we age, homocysteine levels are generally expected to increase and additional amounts of folic acid as well as other B vitamins should be increased proportionately to meet the elderly patient's needs.

As you might have noticed, the phrase "even mildly" has appeared in many of the study reports we have just cited. It suggests a contrary view to the current reference ranges and reports they only identify a risk at levels of 14-15.

## SUMMARY

Elevated homocysteine is a contributor to heart disease and stroke and has also been implicated in Alzheimer's, dementia and damaged DNA. What the medical profession has permitted as acceptable "safe ranges" may actually be far from safe, and only those tested would know their true "at-risk" status. Bile acid sequestrant drugs like Colistid (Colestipol) assigned to many patients for the purpose of lowering cholesterol have an ability to bind folate, thereby enabling a pathway for increased homocysteine levels. These patients would probably benefit from being closely monitored, as would those who are prescribed the popular arthritis drug methotrexate, which also inhibits the first enzyme in a chain that would, in the final analysis, result in a negative interaction with folate. Many arthritis patients remain on this drug for indefinite periods of time. Most assuredly, patients taking higher doses of nicotinic acid (as niacin or niaspan) should be tested to learn what amounts of supplements are necessary to counteract the inverse interaction between niacin and homocysteine. Note: It was not learned until late in the research that a German study found the drug fenofibrate also raised homocysteine levels 44%. Vitamins B6, B12 and folate were found effective in controlling the adverse levels. Based on the evidence, homocysteine qualifies as one of the "silent hidden killers." It may only be a matter of time before national guidelines are modified to encourage maintenance of even lower levels than are accepted by today's standards.

# Chapter 18

# Bypass Surgery
## *Complications*

*M*ental deterioration has been a concern with 30-80% of
bypass patients. Many of these patients experience temporary mental consequence, but the real extent of the potential
permanent damage was not totally understood until very recently, when the longer studies were completed.

## IDENTIFYING THE PROBLEM

During *by-pass*, the patient is totally dependent upon
the heart and lung machine, as the heart and lung functions are taken over by the apparatus. As blood pressure is
lowered for long periods of time, patients often experience
additional drops in their blood pressure, depriving their
brains of adequate oxygen. It is here also that the treatment of blood clotting becomes an even greater concern.
Fortunately many patients who undergo this procedure
display none of these negative symptoms, however, certain patients are exposed to greater risk of later experiencing

mental deterioration, changes in their personality and decline in their ability to think abstractly. Certain study findings assign the blame to the prolonged periods a patient remains under *anesthesia*. The elderly patient is particularly susceptible. Many of these risk factors are reduced in the *minimally invasive* or "**keyhole**" surgeries, which permit the physician to operate on a *beating heart*. But alas, even this surgery has its own set of risks. Not everyone is a candidate for this technique. For those who qualify, even five-way by-pass procedures have been done successfully.

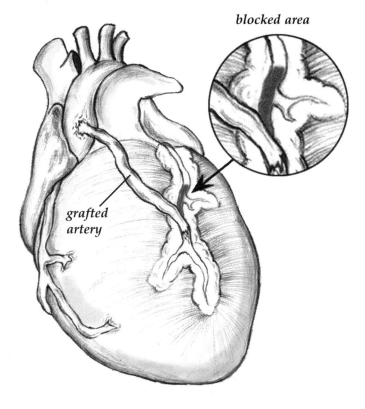

Fig 3: Artery bypass graft

# THE MESSAGE: DON'T REQUIRE BY-PASS!

**Preventive measures you are reading about are directed at saving you from the need to experience by-pass surgery. Please take this information to heart!**

Now is the time to identify and rectify abnormalities that could cause you to ever need this dramatic, invasive surgery. The answer lies in PREVENTION. There is an FDA approved procedure, which we will discuss, that is successfully administered to certain patients who either don't want by-pass or who are not candidates for it.

## ALL IS NOT GOLD

Two new studies have been performed in an attempt to arrive at a better understanding of post-bypass surgery's causes of mental deterioration in the areas of *cognitive mental function*. Areas studied involve the patient's ability to concentrate, to remember, and the degree of the their general mental impairment. Surveys have shown that the patient's own relatives often indicate that the person that they knew seemed somehow changed—a phenomenon that may often go unmentioned in pre-op discussions. Nonetheless, bypass surgery is a proven lifesaving procedure.

However, one *needs* to be cognizant of the risks, and hopefully elect to take the diagnostic journey to prevention long before having to consider this drastic course of action.

One of the two studies emanated from *Johns Hopkins* and the other from *Duke University*. Dr. Mark Newman, the Duke University study author, in an interview with *National Public Radio*, presented five-year statistics on memory, concentration, attention and *manual dexterity* compromise among the test subjects following bypass surgery.

> The mystery doctors have previously been wrestling with is why so many of their patients have experienced dramatic decline in their mental state several years <u>after</u> their surgery.

It was learned from the studies that many of these patients had actually shown an improvement in cognitive mental functions in the immediate weeks and months following the surgeries. These studies were developed to find out why these same patients go on to experience decline in the following years and why this phenomenon even occurs.

**After five years of following 200 patients (with 172 subjects completing the five years), the Duke study concluded that <u>42%</u> of the patients showed significant deterioration in the same skills and abilities that they had been tested for prior to surgery.**

According to Dr. Mark Newman from the Duke study, as published in the February 2001 *New England Journal of Medicine*, 20% of the patients studied had shown a decline in function. The doctor explained in the interview that the amount of decline might show itself in one's lessened manual dexterity and loss of function with regard to speed and memory. The researchers, in quantifying the patient's actual degree of mental decline, determined the amount by comparing the patients' post-op skills to the rate of decline non-bypass patients would be expected to *show over a twenty year span of time.* The researchers sought to determine what rate of decline for non-bypass subjects would be considered average over the twenty year period between 40 and 60 years of age, compared to the difficulties actual open-heart surgery patients would experience following their surgery. Very specifically, they studied how simple tasks became complicated chores. The test areas would be *memory, concentration* and *attention.* An analogy was offered by the reporting doctor, who compared the situation to a right-handed person's difficulty in having to adjust to using their left hand, or vice versa. Reasons for the progressive dysfunction (as explained by Dr. Newman) resulted from the following factors.

**Dislodgement of small particles of plaque that loosened during the actual surgery, only to complete their migration to a vital organ years later** *eventually blocking vessels to the patient's brain and impairing normal mental functions.* Another possibility mentioned was that a significant drop in blood pressure during surgery might have damaged the brain.

## THE FIGHT TO FIX THE HEART AND LUNG MACHINE PROBLEM

Now that the problem has been identified—and **the statistics clearly show a 42% decline in regard to mental acumen among heart and lung patients**—the profession is moving to find ways to lessen the risk exposure during this life saving surgery. According to Cardio-thoracic surgeon Dr. Douglas Boyd, associated with the *London Health Sciences Center* and reported in ABC News:

*"There is clear evidence that neurological damage occurs after the use of the heart and lung machine," and cannot be ignored by anyone in the field of heart surgery."*

One method being studied, for improving the outcome of the surgery according to Favaro's report, is to implant a temporary filter at the aorta (the largest artery in the coronary tree). The idea is to filter tiny bits of plaque that may have broken loose at the site of the heart and lung machine's connection to the artery. Another method being used is to cool the body, working under the assumption that elevated temperatures endanger the process and contribute to more complications.

## MEDICAL MISDIAGNOSIS AND ERROR

Have you ever had the unpleasant experience of driving out of an auto shop only to find that even though the car spent two days in the service bay, the same problem that brought you to the mechanic in the first place was still there? Not to mention the fact that when you drove off, your wallet was lighter by $450. Misdiagnosis also happens very often in medicine. Resident physicians at medical schools and learning hospitals give hands-on training to interns, asking each of them, as they make the rounds, for their interpretation of the symptoms of a particular cooperating patient. The instructing physician may get five or six different diagnoses based on the same criteria. Only one of these diagnoses is the correct one. Mistakes in medicine can, and do happen.

Consider also that the practice of medicine is not a science; it is more correctly characterized as an art. One practices "the art of medicine." Practice makes perfect! One doctor's evaluation may not have revealed a thing to worry about in a certain patient, but another would have seen the warning signs and moved to avoid a negative final outcome. Medical error happens much more often than you might care to know about. A recent national magazine claimed that between 44,000 and 98,000 patients a year die from misdiagnosis and medical error.

> **Put a paintbrush in the hands of two different artists with the same educational background and their work would be quite dissimilar. Give two different doctors the same patient and they may very well come up with two opposing diagnoses.**

Hence the need for second opinions.

## THE FUTURE IS HERE

There is a form of *Angiothensis*, which was mentioned earlier, being developed in a revolutionary and very promising gene therapy approach called *vascular endothelial growth factor* (VEGF). This amazing promising technology in late 2001 lost its leading pioneer and proponent, Dr. Jeffrey Isner, M.D., who in the prime of his effort became a victim *of all things,* a heart attack. According to the earliest reports, the institutions experimenting and developing this gene therapy have been cataloging some remarkable results. One researcher told me (off the record) that if he were an oncologist and being asked about a cure for cancer, he would have to say in regard to (VEGF): "I think we might have found it." Gene therapy may one day in the very near future provide a viable alternative to open heart surgery for many patients.

## AN ALTERNATIVE TO BYPASS

There is another FDA approved procedure that in effect accomplishes angiothensis in yet another way. It was presented at the American Heart Association's Sessions *meeting in Anaheim CA in 2001 and is called Enhanced External Counterpulsation* (EECP). The process is not difficult to explain. For the right candidate, it is a simple solution to a very complex problem. Patients suffering from angina, chest pain, and symptomatic shortness of breath are not receiving the proper amount of blood and oxygen to areas of the heart. Bypass surgery or angioplasty was obviously developed to open or circumvent those arteries that are the source of the problem. EECP provides an extremely low-risk alternative to these invasive procedures.

## HOW EECP WORKS

It is one of the newest procedures gaining popular support, but the concept was discovered close to 51 years ago at *Harvard Medical.* At first look, it seems almost too easy to be a true alternative to bypass surgery. The procedure uses blood pressure-type cuffs that are placed around the patient's legs and thighs. The compressions applied through these cuffs, through inflation and deflation, are timed electronically to coincide with the patient's exact heartbeat.

The interval that the heart relaxes between beats is timed to the exact instant the pressure is applied. Blood is forced upward from the lower body to the heart. **The final result will be the forced formation of "collateral" vessels around occluded arteries**—a *"natural bypass."* As the heart continues its natural beat, the pressure from the cuff is released, which relieves the pressure to the heart and in turn lowers the blood vessel resistance in the patient's legs. Patients often sleep through the 35 one-hour sessions. Some patients prefer doubling up their sessions and finishing within 17 days. From the earliest reports, it appears that EECP may be one of the most viable alternatives for patients unable or unwilling to undergo bypass surgery. It may be a procedure you might discuss with your doctor if you are considering bypass or suffering severe angina. Centers administering EECP are opening across the country and claiming as much as 80% improvement among recipients of the procedure.

# Chapter 19

# *Gum Disease*
## *Linked to* Heart Disease

There have been several studies to determine if in fact gum disease, often called *gingivitis* as the commercials on television have educated us, is yet another villain in the heart disease saga. Gum disease is referred to by several names: periodontal disease, peridontitis, gingivitis, or most commonly, *swollen "bleeding gums"* and involves the bacterium *Porphyromonas gingivalis.*

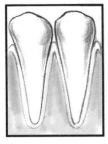 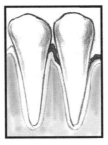 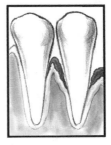

Normal      Beginning stage      Advanced

**Fig 4: The stages of gingivitus**

Most of the time, the public views gum disease as a *minor* concern, and do not know the serious health implications of this ailment and its involvement in building of plaque in the arteries. It has been believed by a good deal of the public that gum disease only became a real source of concern when teeth began to loosen, but studies in recent years have taught that the situation is much more complicated. *Example*: An individual who has gum disease has a 25% increased risk of heart disease over someone with healthy gums. Further study results were made public by Dr. Tiejian Wu and his associates at the State University of New York in Buffalo, New York. Their study, indicated an even stronger relationship between gum disease and two other inflammatory markers we have discussed, **fibrinogen** and **C-reactive protein**. This study enrolled some 10,000 participants. Here is another example of how more than one factor complicates the patient's at-risk patient profile.

*Smoking, is believed to be the root cause of fifty percent of gum disease in the general adult population.* The study, which appeared in the *Journal of Periodontology* included 12,000 adults.

> Those who smoked less than a half pack per day were still almost three times more likely than non-smokers to have periodontal disease. Those who smoked more than a pack and a half per day had almost SIX TIMES THE RISK!

This, according to Drs. Scott Tomar and Sarnira Asma researchers at the *Centers for Disease Control and Prevention,* (CDC) in Atlanta, Georgia.

# A CONFIRMING STUDY

How common is periodontal disease, and who is at heightened risk of developing or worsening heart disease progression? A study presented at the *American Heart Association's* yearly meeting produced some very strong statistical findings. When Dr. Efthymios Deliargyris (with North Carolina, Chapel Hill) along with his associates compared a cross-section of 38 recent heart attack victims with exactly the same number of non-heart attack subjects, they found that 85% of the heart attack recipients had periodontal disease. This is another reason to have yourself tested for the C-reactive protein marker to identify if there is ongoing infection. Those people who grind or clench their teeth during sleep damage the surface of the teeth but the pressure also translates to irritation of the underlying gums causing them to inflame, bleed and subsequently loosen.

According to the *American Academy of Periodontology,* genetics will play a 30% role in increased susceptibility to the disease. We all know that stress in our daily lives from finances, work, relationships or other sources weakens the immune system making one susceptible to gum disease.

Diabetics in general have a greater propensity toward infections, and periodontal disease is no exception. Diabetic patients must be particularly monitored. *Gum disease is a manageable ailment but it requires definite careful attention.* The combined evidence displaces the notion that one need only see the dentist when a toothache occurs. Most people are not aware of the serious nature of gum disease. It might be helpful if the link to heart disease were specifically included in oral hygiene discussions. Frequent dental cleanings and proper oral hygiene is still the best prevention of this disease. Incidentally, it is bacterial *plaque* the dentist is removing during the cleaning procedure.

## STROKE RISK VISIBLE IN DENTAL X-RAYS

Apparently a dentist studying 360 degree panoramic view X-rays of their patient might find something even more significant than dental problems. So says Dr. Arthur Friedlander, an oral and maxillofacial surgeon, and his associate vascular surgeon Dennis Baker of the Veterans hospital in Los Angeles. In studying dental X-rays of 295 men whom had not previously presented with stroke symptoms or events, ten individuals were identified with having visible calcification in the neck (carotid) arteries. Nine of the ten men were smokers. Eighty five thousand people die each year because plaque is released from the carotid arteries.

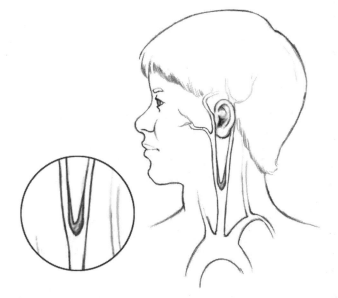

Fig 5: Carotid artery plaque

If calcification is noted in an individual during such exams, the patient is referred to a cardiologist to begin rigorous treatment with statin, fibrate or possibly niacin drugs. The total number of overall stroke deaths annually is around 150,000. Your dentist may not think to interpret this factor when viewing your x-rays—remind him to please do so.

## SUMMARY

Periodontal disease is a product of a bacterial infection and plays a contributing role in atherosclerosis as do the other infections we are addressing including helicobacter pylori and chlamydia pneumonaie. Besides the obvious discomfort of sensitive gums, there is an associated foul breath, as well as the loss of the bone which surrounds and holds the teeth. Unattended, this process leads to the eventual loss of the teeth themselves. There is little disagreement as to the risk of gum disease generating or accelerating one's heart disease.

*THE REMEDY . . .*

▶ Frequent proper brushing and flossing

▶ Frequent oral rinse with an antiseptic mouthwash such as *Listerine* or one recommended by the dentist.

▶ More frequent visits to the dentist for cleaning and observation. *Twice a year (particularly among elder patients) may not be enough to monitor and treat this disease.*

▶ Your dentist may find it necessary to plane and scrape the underlying bone to arrest the degeneration.

▶ A CRP blood test. You may need to insist on the test to learn the level of the infection. Many dentists will not yet be aware of the importance of CRP and heart disease risk.

▶ A possible antibiotic treatment by your dentist to fight the inflammation.

▶ Addition of Coenzyme Q10 if you are not already including it for the heart benefit. (CoQ10 has been found in many studies to aid dramatically in treatment of gum disease).

▶ Supplement of vitamin C.

The disease *scurvy* is a disease sailors on their way to the new world discovered centuries ago when citrus and vitamin C were absent from their diets. A deficiency in this vitamin with the accompanying symptoms of excessive bleeding and gum retraction, is remedied by vitamin C intake. There have also been studies which confirm a connection to heart valve damage resulting from teeth that have become abscessed as well as from advanced gum disease.

# Chapter 20

# 50,000 people per year die *"routinely"*

## *from infections acquired in the hospital*

*H*ere *is yet another reason why preventive care and education is so critically important.* This is why we should try to avoid a need for hospital procedures and those "routine" surgeries if possible. Whenever somebody goes under anesthesia to be operated on, there is risk. No one can disregard the real possibility of contracting a *staph* infection. According to CDC statistics, 260,000 patients in American hospitals will acquire Staphylococcus aureus bacteria ("staph") each year. The amount of patients who die from infections contracted during hospital stays is alarming. As if the staph germ we have been dealing with in this country all these years isn't bad enough, there is a new strain that has migrated from Japan, first recognized in May of 1997. It is another case of a "super bug." Officials from the Centers of Disease Control and Prevention have been working overtime to try and isolate this particular drug resistant strain. The CDC knew this strain would eventually migrate from Asia; it was not whether or not it would make the journey, but simply how soon. Could a drug be made available to counter it? The antibiotic drug *Vancomycin* has been used as a last ditch effort to treat all staph infections. It has been fairly effective until recently, with the emergence of the Japanese strain. The CDC has said that over-prescription of this last ditch antibiotic may be the problem that has created this new drug-resistant monster. It has been said that medicine has **one drug left in the arsenal**. Has medicine fired all its bullets? Pharmaceutical companies are working very hard to see that other drugs are made available to join in the battle against the "super bugs." Two of the newer drugs are *Zyvox* and *Synercid*. But still there are rising fears among infectious disease specialists like Dr. Stuart Levy of *Tufts University Medical School* of Boston. The doctor, in a report appearing in the *Wall Street Journal*, referred to the vancomycin-resistant bacterial infection as **"the one we're afraid of."**

## SUPERBUGS!

Perhaps the greatest infection risk today is from antibiotic-resistant staph infections like *Methicillin-resistant* staph aureus (MRSA), which may present an even greater risk than the surgery itself! Dr. Tim Naimi, medical epidemiologist for *The Center for Disease Control and Prevention*, has said that this MRSA is not new and has been prevalent in hospitals for decades. The situation now, however, is new and different. "The resistance gene may have evolved over a long period of time," according to Dr. Naimi, "protecting the bacteria from many types of commonly used antibiotics such as *penicillin* and *cephalosporins*." We **are** dealing with an invasion of the **"super-bugs"**. It would not be accurate to say that *methicillin-resistant staph aureus* is restricted to hospitals and long-term facilities where it has always been found. On the contrary, according to a report by CDC officials:

> **MRSA has found its way into the community outside the hospital setting and is now regarded by the CDC as an emerging, community-acquired infection. The center is concerned that it might become widespread in certain areas of the US.**

This drug-resistant form of staph claimed the lives of four children in Minnesota and North Dakota. There are **500,000 bypass surgeries** being done a year in this country alone, and exposure to staph remains a major threat.

The point remains, staph infection is a bona-fide life-threatening concern for anyone experiencing any surgery. You might consider learning how many cases of staph have been reported from a particular hospital before your surgery. Some hospitals have a very poor infection control record.

## FALLING ON DEAF EARS

Despite all this information out there to warn us not to take our health for granted, and to initiate simple sacrifices to insure our continued good health, there are those who choose another side of the argument. We all have had friends in denial who say things like, "are you nuts? Cut down on my steak and butter? Eat egg beaters and tofu? You gotta be out of your mind! I've been eating this way

for fifty years, you think I'm gonna stop now? Smoking—
why hell my granddad smoked until he was 92 and died
making love!" All this bravado. All this denial. Remember
the TV transmission-shop ad? *Pay now, or pay later!* If you
absolutely have to go through surgery, ok, but if you could
eliminate the need to experience it in the first place by
getting a little more involved with your own healthcare
and taking early preventive measures predicated on timely
diagnosis, wouldn't you, and shouldn't you? We do have a
choice.

One wonders if sometimes doctors aren't a little too
accommodating in appeasing their patients for fear of
losing or offending them. "Sam, your cholesterol is getting
just a wee bit high, this 265 doesn't look toooo good Sammy,
could you maybe cut down a little on the fats and exercise
just a little more?" More? Sam hasn't been off the couch in
ten years and the only "more" exercise he would do is if
someone moved the refrigerator out on the service porch
or out in the garage. He hasn't seen his feet in at least five
years and has no intention of changing anything. It's been
said, "cancer cures smoking and heart attacks cure lifestyle."
Maybe a direct approach would be more beneficial to the
patient. "Sam, I can't save you if you won't cooperate. My
time with my patients who want to be helped is far too
limited as it is. Perhaps the best way I can help you pro-
long your life is to tell you to either get your ass on a diet or
find a new doctor!" Earlier this year a doctor (Frederick
Ross in Winnepeg, Canada) actually did a similar thing.
He informed his patients that if they didn't want to stop
smoking, they would need to find another doctor. Point
made?

## THE MESSAGE: EARLY PREVENTIVE CARDIOLOGY TO AVOID MAJOR SURGERY

A patient's overall cardiovascular risk status would be less a mystery to their doctors if their individual risk factors were known. Consider a patient in mid-life experiencing severe chest pain, or having suffered an out-and-out heart attack. These arterial blockages didn't just suddenly form overnight. They had been building like debris in a stream for years.

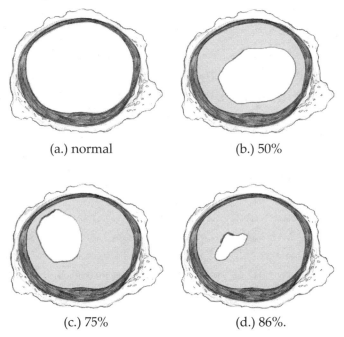

(a.) normal                    (b.) 50%

(c.) 75%                       (d.) 86%.

**Fig 6: Stages of arterial blockage**

**A heart attack that strikes someone in their forties, fifties or sixties is a check that had actually been written 4, 5, or 6 decades earlier only to be cashed at this late date.**

To say the doctor's first awareness of this disease comes when the patient is falling off the treadmill or can no longer negotiate a five-minute walk is ludicrous. Today, with the new EBCT noninvasive CT heart scan, a physician can learn that their patient had been accumulating arterial calcification. If it is discovered early, steps can be implemented to change the course of the disease years before a cardiovascular event announces the earth shattering news: guess what, you have *advanced* heart disease! In effect, all of these tests provide the physician a roadmap as to the individual patient's inherited risk factors. For example, medical science now understands there are different components that make up an individual's LDL and HDL cholesterol.

## SUBCLASS DYSFUCTION HIDES WITHIN ONE'S LDL AND HDL

These subclasses (as they are called) can hide a lot of destructive artery clogging material within their structure. Without exploratory testing, your doctor could not know that your heart disease was developing or progressing **in spite of an arrested LDL score.** These factors, when in dysfunction, can be modified and corrected. How, without testing, would it be recognized that **regardless of total cholesterol** the result could signal the inheritance of a gene that might predispose the patient to a five or six-fold increased chance of heart disease? Unfortunately, the fact is that too few physicians subscribe to the newer information, laboring under the misconception that diet or statin therapy is all that is necessary. Many of today's knowledgeable researchers and physicians would not consider this thinking to be that of a leading edge practitioner in lipid or inflammatory management. In many cases the reason for not testing might be attributable to the fact that the HMO or other insurance company does not want to allocate or approve additional test costs. It would not be unreasonable to suggest that both reasons are involved in the final decision. You just might have to pay the additional expense of $200-$400 yourself.

We both know it is almost beyond the pale to even think about additional health costs when what we are paying for coverage is already unbelievable. Well, if it costs the price of a new DVD for the kids, or a weekend vacation, and it might mean the difference between life and death, isn't it worth it? You are now becoming more informed about what is available for a leading edge evaluation. Is all this getting your attention? It is my intention to bring you, based on the clinical evidence, to that realization. Patients hearing that they have hypertension (elevated blood pressure) probably wouldn't conclude the condition was going to kill them. There was a time, before the advent of modern medicines, when the patient might have been inclined so to conjecture. Wouldn't we agree that today, the advice would be to control one's blood pressure and go on with their life? It would seem that early identification of the total heart disease profile (which we are discussing) should follow the same course. "But I may not want to know." Well, you surely would know *after the heart attack,* or as with other diseases, when blood is found in the bowl possibly indicating an advanced disease that had gone undetected far too long. The outcome might have been quite different if the problem had been found and dealt with much earlier by a "full body" scan or other proactive examination.

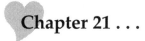

# Chapter 21

# *LP (a)*

## Risk Factor # IV, Inherited

Known as (LP little a) and not to be confused with apolipoprotein (big) A, LP (a) can raise one's heart attack risk as much as five-fold. LP (a) is an inherited risk factor and an even more destructive component of regular LDL "bad" cholesterol which as we already know plays a role in contributing to both atherosclerosis development and stroke risk.

▶ In atherosclerosis, LP (a) binds with fibrin in the formation of arterial plaque.

▶ It creates and carries very sticky fat particles through the blood leading to deadly blood clots. These clots can either be the pathway to a heart attack or a stroke.

In 1994 Linus Paulings had ascertained through his investigation at the *Linus Paulings Institute* that elevations in this inherited trait were **ten times more dangerous than**

**LDL cholesterol.** Various studies have arrived at different findings in regard to dangerous levels. Whether they find the risk of elevations to be 5-7 or 10 times greater, they all agree that higher elevations add a significant risk.

> **The results of the (HERS) study found that women with the highest levels of LP (a) had a 54% greater risk of heart disease.**

There is more about this risk factor in the following case history. A previous illustration presented was labeled *a fictional reality*; the following *non-fictional* illustration is offered similarly to demonstrate what happens when the new science is translated from diagnostic discovery into actual application. LP (a) has been implicated in the development of peripheral artery disease and particularly **carotid disease.** Peripheral disease takes a toll in *the legs* as well as the *carotid arteries* in the neck leading to the brain. These arteries, like the coronary arteries can also become "narrowed" with plaque buildup. Clot formations in the carotids pose an ever-present threat of *"brain attack."* Plaque dislodgement from the leg can also migrate to the lung.

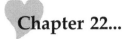 Chapter 22...

# An Actual
# *Recent Case History*

## APPLYING THE NEW INFORMATION

The following case provides a tangible illustration of how the new information identified multiple contributing disorders in one particular patient's profile that had eluded the "normally accepted" screening techniques for decades. Do you know if you have any of these disorders complicating your heart attack and stroke profile or that of your spouse?

This subject individual has had a long, protracted history of heart disease. She was fortunate enough to have had a very fine team of surgeons attending her surgeries as interventions to treat advancing peripheral artery disease became warranted. One of these procedures, an *endarterectomy*, was performed to clear a more than 85% obstruction of the carotid artery.

The outcome was successful, however *the actual overall inherited and inflammatory heart disease factors still*

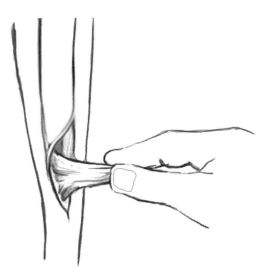

Fig 7: Carotid plaque

*remained unidentified even after surgery. Her primary physicians for the three years prior had not treated her cholesterol and it now was at an incredible 315 with a runaway LDL of 215, 115% over what it should be given her history.*

Two years after the carotid surgery it became necessary for the patient to undergo yet another independent invasive procedure. It is important to note that each of the *two procedures the patient underwent were performed to intercede against the progression of advancing <u>peripheral artery disease</u> (PAD).* **LP (a) is one of the major contributors to this form of heart disease and would be revealed in this patient's positive LP (a) test result.**

**Of the many reported studies was one in which Oxford scientists determined that elevated LP (a) had been responsible for** increasing heart attack risk over a ten year period by 70%.

## PATIENT'S SECOND SURGERY

This patient's second procedure necessitated the insertion of two stents, one in each leg to rectify advanced obstruction. *Obvious multi-vessel peripheral disease, whose actual contributing sources had never been identified and treated were allowed to persist since the earlier surgery.* Not only had the carotid and major coronary arteries been affected by the combination of dysfunctions, but now the femoral arteries in the legs had also occluded. This patient's pulse was barely audible in the left arm because of almost total stenosis of the artery supplying blood to this extremity attributable to the advanced degree of disease. In addition, yet another coronary artery was also almost totally occluded. As was explained to the patient, the reason she was able to function in spite of all the compromised arterial flow was that her body had developed arterioles, *or "collateral vessels,"* as they are sometimes called. These smaller vessels provide a natural bypass around blocked arteries. **Here is the point of presenting and including all of this patient's history**: the obvious effects of this patient's disease (not uncommonly) were being treated with interventional surgery as the effects warranted.

## UNDETECTED CAUSES

**The actual *causes* were never explored or identified by any of the four primary care physicians who had attended this individual.** Is it possible they were not aware or had not realized the import of the information? As a consequence, the patient's inherited and acquired risk factors were not identified, and a destructive process went on unabated. Certainly, the results of one physician's work or approach, when compared to the scrutiny of another, may produce a quite different outcome. I suggested to this patient that she discuss with a doctor having the inherited risk factors analyzed. The information acquired from this exploration, I dare say, will demonstrate the benefit of exploring and identifying a heart patient's underlying "hidden" heart risks and provide yet another example of why second opinions are advisable.

> Doctors agree in their admirable ethical oath to *do no harm;* however, there are times in certain situations when simply doing too little diagnostically, may actually cause <u>more</u> harm to the very patient the doctor is trying to help.

To further exacerbate the health of this particular patient, a blocked artery had been regurgitating blood from a *diseased calcified mitral heart valve* — a valve condition which, when advanced, may actually cause the reversal of blood flow through the coronary artery. This occurs as the normal direction of flow is rejected by the advanced accumulation of calcium of the aortic or in this case mitral valve. There are of course other diseases that also affect heart valves. An EBCT scan no doubt would have warned of this advancing calcification process many years earlier.

## READING THE TEA LEAVES

**The following interpretation** illustrates how the new information might translate from identification to treatment of the root cause of the development and advancement of disease. It is not presented as a *"cut-in-stone"* scientific interpretation, but rather as an example of how the newer test results can be interpreted and benefit derived. While the *Berkeley HeartLab* itself is available to provide doctors and patients with an analysis of a patient's test results and suggestions for a formulated plan of treatment, *what you are about to read would not necessarily be their interpretation, and must not be assumed to be such.* It is, however, an interpretation based on clinical science and trial findings, and that collective information suggests the following conclusions:

## THE PATIENT'S RESULTS, TEST A

The patient was tested for several risk factors and proved to have very high previously undetected scores on *four* of the tests. The fourth test for C-reactive protein (which had not been initially requested) was performed in early 2001 with an alarming dysfunctional result, as you will see. One of the original tests, as you might expect, would be a test for LP (a).

> The LP (a) trait (depending on one's score) can actually increase one's heart attack risk by as much as *five times.*

If you are concerned with heart disease (or someone you know is), this LP (a) gene should be tested and most definitely if there has been family history of heart disease.

## TWO AND HALF TIMES NORMAL

An LP (a) score of 5 is accepted on reference range scales as ideal and 10 and above enters the range of concern with above 25 mg/dl as being very high. This particular patient's profile we are reviewing presented a score of **35, two and a half times beyond the "acceptable" range!** Severe elevation in this gene score is a direct source of carotid and peripheral artery disease affecting the legs and neck arteries. Based on the clinical evidence and a pound of common sense, should there be any wonder that this patient's symptomatic conditions had progressed to the point of interventional carotid surgery as well as the second procedure to open both leg arteries? A good number of cardiologists and physicians would agree that highly elevated LP (a) would have to be considered a contributing factor particularly when viewed along with the very high accompanying LDL score. A patient should not have to learn they have an inherited heart risk (250%) beyond optimum so late in the game, particularly when there was something that could be done to inhibit the risk if the dysfunction had been earlier detected. The time for finding the root cause of an individual's heart disease is early in life. There is no need to watch and wait while unaltered and uninterrupted progression brings the patient to eventual crisis or even death and yet that is the way heart disease has been managed until now. There would still prove to be additional undesirable test results found in this patient's profile complicating the entire spectrum.

## PATIENT'S TEST B

An *electrophoresis* study was done, and the patient was determined to be an apolipoprotein type "B". An indication small, dense LDL particles were rapidly entering the bloodstream and adhering to the artery walls. Niacin, along with a statin drug, would reduce this dysfunction as well as the high LP (a) value significantly.

## PATIENT'S TEST C

This patient would also be evaluated for the bacterial infection chlamydia pneumoniae. Inflammation at the arterial wall involves the endothelium, the smooth cell structure that lines the arteries. As we have learned, the endothelium, when inflamed or otherwise injured, is a breeding ground for the development of atherosclerosis. In short, inflammation within the arteries is never a "good thing." As we have suggested, inflammation is the *new frontier of cardiovascular research,* and many conditions that increase inflammatory response are under investigation. One of the paramount concerns in regard to heart attack and stroke is the role played by an adverse relationship between bacterial, viral infections and vulnerable or "unstable plaque."

## THE Cp TEST RESULTS

The subject patient's results for this inflammatory C pneumonie test also proved positive, with an IgG score of 1:53. Three years later, without the infection having been treated, the score would be recorded as 1:63. The testing had now uncovered **this second risk factor, which had not been detected in the patient's prior blood evaluations. Remember the statistic that "80% of these inherited risk factors would not be found during routine blood work?"** For all intents and purposes, there is no indication that the identified infection or the LP (a) gene would ever have been detected without these newer tests. The patient had also presented with an exceptionally high LDL and total cholesterol value which in combination with the other out-of-line risk mechanisms, would only complicate the heart disease risk profile and hasten the destructive course of this individual's overall heart disease.

## PATIENT'S TEST D, C-REACTIVE PROTEIN

**The patient's score for C-reactive protein (CRP), would be discovered to be *extremely* high at 8.3!**

You may recall the CRP findings presented earlier from the work of *Dr. Paul Ridker* from Harvard, whose study found a *high CRP level among women could amount to an increased heart attack risk of 7.3 times.* In the Harvard *Women's Health Study* many of the women with the higher CRP scores were from families without a previous family history of heart disease. Furthermore, many had normal levels of cholesterol supporting the fact that C-reactive protein is an *independent* risk for heart attack and stroke. In order for a physician to properly evaluate *this* patient's total at-risk profile we are presenting, the test results would need to be studied collectively with particular consideration given to the patient's very high LDL of 215! *Prescribing a cholesterol drug alone, and sending the patient home expecting a miracle, would not be the answer—but we can imagine that is exactly what happens in cases when the patient has not been evaluated for the other risk factors.*

## NEUTRALIZING THE 5 DYSFUNCTIONS

▶ **LP (a)** elevations respond to *Niacin* therapy.

▶ **Chlamydia pneumonaie**, preferred antibiotic treatment *Zithromax*, (azithromycin), *roxithromycin*.

▶ **C-Reactive Protein**, *ASA* (aspirin) reduces CRP 55.7%.

▶ **Apolipoprotein B,** *Niacin* alters the negative status to A.

▶ **LDL and total Cholesterol.** For difficult management cases, a combination of statin drug therapy with niacin or bile acid sequestrant, diet and exercise.

All of this information is based on the study findings of physicians, scientists and researchers in the field of cardiology, and may help you in discussion with your own doctor. Hopefully, presenting this one patient's case history has given you a better understanding of how this lifesaving information can be applied. The full spectrum of risk must be evaluated and controlled. Now, HAVING READ ALL OF THIS, recall the examples we discussed in the book's opening chapter of the **ice skater and the golfer** who died of heart attacks **and the man** who expired on his doctor's steps at the clinic. Could the tests discussed here have saved patient's lives—possibly? Could these tests have raised red flags revealing the *hidden risk factors* in time for their physician to implement steps of intervention? Yes, more than likely. Perhaps more importantly, would these individuals and their respective physicians have known specifically what they were dealing with instead of helplessly awaiting the inevitable? Most assuredly, emphatically, yes! You may be wondering why these newer tests to find the "hidden risks" aren't currently administered to a patient as a matter of course during a routine physical, even if only occasionally. Why not use all of the available protocols and preventive information available to save something as irreplaceable as someone's father or other family member? Perhaps you are questioning whether we are overly concerned with heart attacks? Please consider how serious the situation is according to the *American*

*Heart Association.* The answer would seem to lie within the following statistics. You could actually hang your hat on this one fact: **"50% of all heart attacks and stroke occur among people with normal cholesterol."** We have studied such risk factors as homocysteine, C-reactive protein and briefly, LP (a); we will explore many more.

## A NON-DRUG CHOLESTEROL FIGHTER!

One non-drug being sold for cholesterol lowering goes by the name *Cholestin,* there are other similar cholesterol-lowering compounds like *Cholestatin* and *Chitosan* (from shellfish) that have shown outstanding results in limited trials. This particular compound (cholestin) is made from a *red yeast* extract of fermented rice. It is actually the ingredient that one sees on Peking Duck. It is what gives this delicacy its color. An in depth study would find that Mevacor (Lovestatin), which is one of the earliest of the statin group of drugs, utilizes *chione* as one of its key ingredients. Chione is derived from Chinese red yeast rice. The following are the study results that were presented at the American Heart Association's 39th *Annual Conference on Cardiovascular Disease Epidemiology and Prevention* in Florida. They are impressive.

The study consisted of 233 elderly participants. These participants were given the AHA's *(American Heart Association's)* Step 1 diet. This is a diet designed for those with normal cholesterol ingesting a limit of 30% of calories from fat. At the end of one month the reported results confirmed zero depreciation of cholesterol levels.

These same individuals when given *Cholestin* orally in pill form for a period of two months demonstrated a 16% decrease in total cholesterol levels, a 21% decrease in LDL "bad guys" and a HDL increase of 14.6%. This study was conducted by *Tufts University School of Medicine* under the direction of Dr. James Rippe. The AHA urged caution in using the condiment, saying: *"Because there are no long-term studies that show red yeast rice to be as safe as diet and/or cholesterol-lowering drugs, the AHA urges individuals with elevated blood cholesterol levels to consult with their physician before introducing cholestin into a cholesterol-lowering regimen."*

This warning should be considered good advice by anyone taking any of the non-drug alternatives. Does this product or the other over-the-counter supplements provide an alternative for those who cannot afford insurance to buy prescription drugs? Time will tell; after all, these study results are short-term numbers and percentages, albeit pretty impressive. A second study was undertaken by the manufacturer *Pharmanex, Inc.* in China, directed by a Dr. Joseph Chang. The results continued to be impressive. The report claimed that of the trial subjects with elevated cholesterol who took *cholestin,* 92% showed some improvement in their levels. *"Cholestin* reduced LDL by 32.8% and decreased triglycerides 19.9%," reported Dr. Chang.

> It is interesting that China has produced two natural substances, green tea and red yeast rice, that seem to offer major benefit in prevention of both cancer <u>and</u> heart disease. Neither is under the control of the American Medical Association, but then nor are chondroitin sulfate, glucosamine, folic acid, MSM, or for that matter vitamins E or C.

# Chapter 23

# Life-affecting Benefits of Tea You Haven't Heard

A study done in *Rotterdam* involving some 3,454 subjects claimed that people could significantly reduce their risk of atherosclerosis simply by drinking two cups of tea daily. How much reduction? Try a 46% reduction of atherosclerosis and plaque formation found in the coronary arteries among those drinkers of just two cups daily, according to Dr. Johanna M. Geleijnse and her research team.

**The study claimed that those individuals with *severe* atherosclerosis whose arteries were examined for coronary plaque actually lowered their risk by a whopping 69% when doubling their tea intake to *four cups* a day.**

These results were obtained during two and three year follow-ups of the study's participants. The report was filed in an issue of the *Archives of Internal Medicine.* Another study, led by Dr. D. Sesso from *Brigham and Women's Hospital* and *Harvard Medical School,* Boston, MA, produced similar results. There was a 46% reduction in heart attack risk in tea drinkers compared to non-tea drinkers. In writing the final report the team noted that tea contains flavonoids, which are recognized for their ability to reduce amounts of LDL oxidation. In Japan and China, where large amounts of green tea are ingested daily, the rate of heart disease remains very low. One reason, according to other studies, might be that green tea (besides producing flavonoids) also contains a category of *polyphenols* called *catechins,* which have been shown in studies to actually inhibit the growth of new blood vessels that cancerous tumors depend on for growth. This process is part of a whole new field of study of how tumor growth is fed. Did you know that as a source of antioxidant the *polyphenols* contained in green tea are 100 times more powerful than vitamin C?

## TAKE TEA AND SEE

So significant were these findings that I searched for more studies to support the benefits of regular tea consumption. A study reported in The *American Journal of Epidemiology* in January 1999 concluded, after interviewing a like number of heart attack and non-heart attack victims, that those who drank one or more cups of black tea daily had a 50% lower heart attack risk when compared to those who did not consume tea in their regular daily diet.

## SUMMARY

According to multiple studies, substituting tea for coffee (at least one cup a day) appears to offer some protection against atherosclerosis. Green tea has been found effective in lowering risks associated with stomach, bladder, lung, liver, esophageal and breast cancer. It lowers LDL cholesterol and its antioxidant properties limit damage from oxidation. It has been shown to benefit arterial flexibility and suppleness, affects both LDL & HDL favorably and lowers triglycerides. With regard to stroke, green tea lowers thromboxane, which is implicated in blood clots that lead to stroke. Given the amazing study results regarding tea consumption, it is hard to understand why more people do not substitute tea for coffee unless like myself, they were not aware of the gross benefits. It is also apparent from the studies that there are pure therapeutic advantages to drinking tea—particularly green tea. If you don't enjoy the flavor of green tea or do not wish to drink the suggested daily amounts, capsules of green tea extract are available.

# Chapter 24

# Making The Case
# *Against* **Fibrinogen**

## RISK FACTOR # V

What is fibrinogen and how do you pronounce it? It is pronounced fi-brin-o-gen and scientifically it may be described as a blood protein that becomes converted into fibrin by thrombin when calcium is present. A more practical explanation would be that fibrin is a thread-like substance with an ability to form a *mesh* to collect and hold blood while a wound or rupture is actually sealed. This important process is known as *fibrinogenesis*. When fibrin is mixed with elevated LDL cholesterol, the combination creates a "fibrin foam," forming a catalyst that contributes to the formation of calcification in the arteries. There is another important function involving fibrinogen called *fibrinolysis*, in which the body breaks down small life-threatening fibrous blood clots. Fibrinogen is therefore involved in both the blood clotting and arterial placqing process, and qualifies as a contributor to both heart disease and stroke. More than one study has found that dangerously high fibrinogen may be found in one out of five people. Have you ever been tested?

This word, fibrinogen, this process, *fibrinogenesis*—why have they not been in the forefront of physician awareness? Fibrinogen under normal conditions provides necessary lifesaving coagulation. This protective benefit is what actually prevents us from bleeding to death after sustaining a wound or cut, however, when fibrinogen in higher levels *overcompensates* in its natural coagulation response the results can be disastrous. Fibrinogen rushes to the rescue; not unlike the way collagen comes to the scene to repair damage. It is here that fibrin is employed to help seal microscopic fissures at the artery wall. Over time the process of "hemorrhage and repair" continues. The assault is repeatedly perpetrated on the endothelium cells at the wall's surface. Permanent atheroclerotic damage is the cumulative result, leading to hardening of the arteries and general heart disease. While it is not yet an opinion universally embraced by physicians who have not kept up with the science, there is overwhelming corroborative evidence that high fibrinogen has indeed been a little understood major risk factor. What you are about to read may arguably be the most involved presentation on the subject of fibrinogen and the case against it being made available to an unsuspecting public.

## THE COURT IS IN SESSION

Fibrinogen, according to a study in 1990 by Nigel Cook and David Ubben, entitled *Fibrinogen as a major cardiovascular risk factor in cardiovascular disease,* suggested that fibrinogen is in fact integrated in **vascular lesions** and is involved in the earliest development of plaque. Appearing before the *18th International Joint Conference on Stroke and Cerebral Circulation*, Dr. Dennis P. Briley proffered that *fibrinogen* concentrations **are also a <u>stronger predictor</u> of the extent of carotid artery stenosis than what one could assign to the <u>*nine*</u> other stroke and cerebral attack criteria.** Are these findings not amazing?

> **Consider that of 140 stroke victims in the study, those whose carotid arteries with a stenosis of less than 50% had fibrinogen levels of 370 mg/dl. In comparison, the study subjects who when tested by ultrasound were found to have a 50-89% blockage, had fibrinogen levels of 403 mg/dl. Even more conclusive, those patients with a major 89% occlusion had shown a total fibrinogen test result of 458 mg/dl.**

Why are so many trials by respected researchers only now just beginning to come forward with vital information concerning this blood protein? Why now, almost four decades after the landmark *Framingham Heart Study* alerted the medical community of this blood protein's role in heart disease and stroke? By the end of this chapter it will be apparent that fibrinogen's time for test evaluation and monitoring has come. A report also illuminated still another negative association between *hypertension* (high blood pressure) and fibrinogen.

> **Patients with a systolic blood pressure of *>180 mm* *when combined with elevated fibrinogen scores became associated with as much as a 12-fold increase of stroke over those in the population with lower scores.***

Perhaps one reason for the delay is the fact that there has never been a known remedy to combat elevations in fibrinogen. Evidence had emerged around 1950 alerting the profession to the connection of fibrinogen to heart disease. It seemed prudent practice, even then, to at least consider evaluating patients showing symptoms of heart disease. *JAMA (Journal of American Medical Association)* published an article in 1987 entitled *Fibrinogen and Risk of Cardiovascular Disease.* This early article presented certain findings of the *Framingham* Study by Kannel WB, Wolf PA, Castelli WP, D'agostino RB. Researchers and doctors recently looking at the tenth year evaluation of the Framingham Study *confirmed* elevated fibrinogen levels to be a predictor of cardiovascular **disease that should be added to the list of cardiovascular risk factors.**

The *Framingham* study further concluded that high fibrinogen was **comparable with other major risk factors** such as smoking, blood pressure, diabetes and *hematocrit* (blood viscosity). It is now almost 15 years later, and the vast majority of physicians are still not evaluating or even considering their patient's fibrinogen levels. Finally, in 1999, the *American Heart Association* made the following statement concerning fibrinogen as a risk factor. In their recent recommendation, the AHA actually added another dimension to the risk profile by informing physicians that high amounts of Low Density Lipoprotein (LDL) cholesterol AND elevated fibrinogen were <u>specifically a dangerous combination</u>. The denial of earlier claims of fibrinogen's role in the CAD process has not been unlike the way homocysteine's contribution had been previously ignored. The wheels turn slowly, but importantly, attention is beginning to become focused on this acute phase reactant and the risk created by even slightly elevated ranges. There is a long way from a discovery by the research community until action is taken in the practicing office. Fibrinogen tests are not routinely administered during physicals or office visits. They are not even on the radar screen.

> I first became aware of fibrinogen as a potential factor several years ago in 1995 when I asked my physician during an annual physical if he wouldn't mind ordering a fibrinogen test.

The open-minded doctor agreed, but asked out of curiosity, **"Why on earth would you want a fibrinogen test, I've never ordered one for anyone?"** When he phoned with the results a few days later he explained, "You are way off the chart but I don't know what exactly to tell you to do about it." He went on to say that his research did not turn up a remedy to lower fibrinogen. With my score now defined as 461 and necessity being the mother of all invention, the task of finding a remedy, like it or not, would become mine. To have a better idea of what a high number might mean, in regard to risk, keep 461 in mind as you read the following.

## HIGH FIBRINOGEN AND AN 85% RISK OF HEART DISEASE

A 1996 British study ascertained the risk among people with fibrinogen levels within the top one-third of the 200-400 point reference scale (between 350 and 400) to be 85%!

The research team of this five-year study, had been regularly testing the blood levels of fibrinogen among the workers in a British food processing plant before arriving at this 85% determination. These determinant values were established independently of other risk factors. Considering this information, how would my score of 461, (61 points beyond the scale and absolutely beyond the 85% risk range) translate to actual risk? I believe fibrinogen would remain the most probable cause of my extremely high calcification score you read about earlier in Chapter 9, *An Author's Journey*. As is becoming obvious from the amount of information in this chapter, it would be one of the markers I would research intensely. Very little was known or published on this subject at the time.

With my high score now discovered and with no known remedy for high fibrinogen, the search for a drug, or combination of drugs, or supplements, or whatever it would take to arrest this *runaway* fibrinogen level, would have to become my mission. There was no other option, and hopefully the public will benefit from what was found. My 461 score eventually was altered through trial and error to 260! Moreover, it soon became clear that levels accepted as **"normal" may in reality, given the evidence, be abnormally and dangerously high.**

Patients who would record in the highest quartile had a 700% increased risk of hemorrhagic stroke and more than twice the chance of actually dying of stroke. The risks were found to be independent of cardiovascular risks, however, fibrinogen and hypertension were the greatest detrimental combination. *J. Epidemiol Community Health 2002;56 (Suppl I:)* We would all be amazed at how very few physicians are familiar with fibrinogen's other roles including one of age association and the newest assigned role as a stress protein. They have been aware of fibrinogen as an acute phase reactant and would expect rising fibrinogen levels following an incident of bodily infection or an expected temporary increase following a heart attack, stroke or for that matter, even a pregnancy.

Temporary elevated scores would be expected for any number of inflammatory diseases, including liver disease, and other traumatic illness. This rise in level would be expected, transient, and destined to subside in time. This is how fibrinogen's singular role as an *acute phase reactant has* always been understood.

According to the most recent studies, fibrinogen plays several other important roles in the cardiovascular/stroke equation. One, genetic, another in the metabolic syndrome as with Diabetes II—a "stress protein"—rising in response to an individual's stress levels, and also as a co-factor in blood clots and development of arterial plaque. A very busy factor to have gone unacknowledged. As a matter of record, it has been documented since the 1950's that high fibrinogen *(fibrinogenenemia)* also increases dramatically as heart disease advances. There is a theory that in this role as an inflammatory respondent, fibrinogen may actually feed upon itself. None of the accusations are favorable.

## FIBRINOGEN'S INVOLVEMENT
## WITH CALCIFICATION

It wasn't until 2002 that I finally located a study whose results confirmed my earlier assumption and connected the dots between my 461 high level of fibrinogen. Appearing in journal ATVB, 9/2000, pgs. 2167-71, was a new study that concentrated on proving a relationship between fibrinogen and a high degree of calcification.

> It was no longer speculation; fibrinogen was proven
> in this study to have a 95% probability of creating
> calcification.

If one subscribes to the information that has been presented in this chapter on fibrinogen, then it would not be unreasonable to consider that my original 461 fibrinogen score contributed to the high calcification scores recorded on the original EBCT test evaluation.

## FIBRINOGEN AND AORTIC ATHEROSCLEROSIS

Calcification in the aorta is always of major concern. In a study appearing in the *American Journal of Cardiology* Vol 81, issue 3, author Christophe Tribouilloy, M.D., Ph.D, and his team, **after evaluating aortic plaque and fibrinogen, reported a direct association between elevated fibrinogen and the severity of thoracic aortic atherosclerosis.** They concluded fibrinogen to be an independent marker for the severity of thoracic aortic plaque rupture or any other cause of bleeding within an artery. Elevated fibrinogen as well is a determining factor in many cases of *"massive heart attacks."*

## FIBRINOGEN MAY DETERMINE THE ACTUAL SIZE OF A HEART ATTACK OR STROKE

Among the various study results filed in this area was one particularly important to this discussion. JD Sutter and his Amsterdam team in 2001 offered an explanation of a direct relationship between fibrinogen levels and actual myocardial infarction result. *The higher the level of fibrinogen, the larger and more dramatic the size of the clot formation* resulting from the bleeding episode following an angioplasty procedure. *Note*: Even though this study was done on bleeding episodes associated with *angioplasty*, it would certainly not be much of a leap to imagine how heart attack patients with elevated fibrinogen might be exposed to devastating larger occlusive clot formation following a plaque rupture or any cause of bleeding within the artery other than from angioplasty procedures.

## HOW SPECIFIC FIBRINOGEN LEVELS INFLICT DAMAGE IN INDIVIDUAL ARTERIES

Combining the findings of contributing doctors, researchers and scientists as source for their conclusions of how fibrinogen levels actually inflict damage within individual arteries, *Berkeley HeartLab Inc.* quantifies the contribution of fibrinogen to the process of heart disease and stroke based in part on the following information. Elevated fibrinogen levels raise the risk of atherosclerosis when in excess *of 277 mg/dl. This level has been associated with a 2.4 fold increase in coronary events compared to values less than 235 mg/dl (Mennch Jj. et al athero thromb 1994,14 54-59).* The combination of elevated fibrinogen with another CAD risk factor increases risk substantially. For example, subjects with combined elevated fibrinogen and elevated LDL (163 mg/dl) have a 6.1 fold (more than 600%!) higher coronary risk. This combination of Fibrinogen and LDL is another reason why looking at the entire risk profile; cholesterol, genetic, environmental, behavioral and inflammatory risk factors are all a necessary part of heart disease and stroke management.

> **Each increase of 75 mg/dl of fibrinogen increases CAD mortality by 29%!** *(Benderly M at al ATVB 1996, 16.351-356)*

Fibrinogen levels are also associated with peripheral vascular disease as determined by the different values ascertained by an individual's test result. The following determinants indicate what might be the risk ratio in each of the individual arteries. **As you will see, the risk in the coronary arteries is more than 3 1/2 times greater. Fibrinogen scores between (280 mg/dl> and 337 mg/dl) translated to a 2.2 fold risk increase in the carotid (neck) arteries. Femoral arteries (legs) risk was 1.8 times but** *the largest* **risk of 3.6 times or 360% was found in atherosclerotic development identified in the coronary arteries.** (Levenson J et al, *Arterioclerosis, Thrombosis, And Vascular. Biology. 1997,45-50).*

**With this documentation and so many supporting trial results in the record, why are so many doctors remaining in the dark as to the role fibrinogen plays in heart disease? Why are so few fibrinogen tests ordered?**

There is additional information from many leading clinical studies whose results, when viewed together, become more than passively convincing that fibrinogen levels should be taken very seriously, and anyone with even mild cardiovascular disease factors might benefit from being tested. Smokers have an increased concern, with a proven correlation between smoking and fibrinosis. Obese individuals also potentially have elevated fibrinogen and CRP levels as well. There is additional information which continues to support the fact that fibrinogen besides being an acute phase reactant may indeed also be of the genetic (inherited) syndrome.

## STRONGEST PREDICTOR

**"Plasma fibrinogen was the strongest independent predictor of death from coronary disease,"** concluded a trial published in 1992.

> *" We conclude that, in patients with peripheral arterial disease—XLFDP (clotting factor), a measure of ongoing fibrin formation and degradation, is a strong predictor of both disease progression and future coronary risk. "*

The six-year study was reported in the journal *Thrombosis, Haemostasis* in 1992 by study authors, Banerjee A.K., Pearson J., Gilliland E.L., Goss D., Lewis J.D., Stirling Y., Meade T.W. In this particular study, a total of 333 patients with stable *intermittent claudication* at recruitment were followed for six years to determine the risk factors leading to subsequent mortality.

**THE STRONGEST PREDICTOR OF DEATH during the follow-up period was the fibrinogen level.**

Cardiovascular diseases were the underlying cause of death in 78% of the 114 patients who had died. *A minor fibrinogen increase was associated with a nearly two-fold increase in the probability of death within the following 6 years* (the report concluded). These results also provide further evidence for the involvement of fibrinogen in the pathogenesis of arterial and peripheral disease. These studies concentrated on *intermittent claudication,* a condition diagnosed by leg pain when walking which tends to subside when the activity ceases or the extremity is rested. The collective evidence more than suggests that if you or someone you know suffers from these symptoms, fibrinogen levels should be suspect and evaluated.

## 6.1 TIMES INCREASED HEART ATTACK RISK

A combination of elevated fibrinogen with high LDL levels, can mean a 6.1 fold increased risk of cardiovascular disease. The study concentrated on the synergy between these two elements. Even slightly elevated LDL in combination with elevated fibrinogen increases risk by a significant percentage.

> **Many leading scientists and cardiologists share a concern that when a plaque ruptures or bleeds, fibrinogen may be a factor determining the actual size and density of clots that form as a result.**

Here, in many cases, it is determined whether one experiences a minor heart attack or stroke or a more serious, perhaps final event based on the degree of clot formation from an overabundance of this blood protein fibrinogen. The evidence compiled by researchers and many leading cardiologists and scientists has been building a strong case against fibrinogen for many years. Many of these trials, reported in journals, have concentrated on the ongoing fibriogenic process. These trials, when you look at their results in concert, more than suggest that, contrary to accepted theory,

> **FIBRINOGEN IS ALSO INVOLVED IN AN ON-GOING INHERITED DYSFUNCTION AND, THEREFORE, IS NOT JUST AN ACUTE PHASE REACTANT AS HAS BEEN ITS RECOGNIZED ROLE**

There are newer studies that suggest a genetic predisposed link to higher elevations of fibrinogen which if identified early would be a warning sign alerting the patient and physician. At a later stage, these effects contribute directly or indirectly to many heart attacks and cases of *thrombotic* stroke and premature death. A report filed in late 2001 by the *New York Academy of Sciences* by Mp de Maat stated that estimates based on twin studies had suggested the following:

> *"30-50% of the plasma fibrinogen level is genetically determined."*

Has your physician ruled out fibrinogen as a potential factor contributing to your particular heart disease? The following opinion appeared in the *Advances in Lipids Newsletter, Vol. 13.* **Plasma levels of fibrinogen are strongly**

**influenced by genetic factors,** thus there is growing interest in the concept that evaluating fibrinogen levels might identify patients at higher risk for cardiovascular events, and that interventions to lower fibrinogen levels might reduce the risk of clinical events.

Perhaps some of the most revolutionary findings have recently come from the British *Whitehall II Study* which has identified yet the newest role for fibrinogen, that of a responder to stress itself. The *Whitehall* went as far as to define and qualify how fibrinogen levels are influenced and responsive to socioeconomic and work related conditions! If the studies which claim that one in five people might have inherited a dysfunctional gene are indeed accurate, then not knowing where you fit in the odds equation becomes an important diagnostic concern. The implications of the following study support the need for identifying the at-risk patient early.

## THE EDINBURGH ARTERY STUDY

The study authors, in an effort to better understand *haemostatic* (blood clotting factors), including those associated with fibrinogen and its involvement and prediction of progression and eventual deterioration into peripheral artery disease (PAD), began a five-year study.

> **The Edinburgh study enrolled 1,592 men and women and found that elevated fibrinogen levels were present among patients who developed or advanced existing peripheral artery disease (PAD).**

# EVIDENCE ON A GENETIC LINK

*M.D. Francois Cambien,* director of research at the *Institut National de la Sante' et la Recherche Medicale* in Paris France, in offering test results of his study of 565 men, explained still another reason why individuals who smoke have a higher incidence of heart attacks and stroke than those who do not. *The findings suggested that anyone with elevated fibrinogen levels may be at even greater risk if they smoke.* The French study found the following:

**ONE IN FIVE PEOPLE MAY CARRY A MUTATION OF THE FIBRINOGEN GENE IN THEIR SYSTEMS.**

In the *PROCAM* (Prospective Cardiovascular Munster) study, investigating the correlation between LDL cholesterol and fibrinogen, the following was documented:

*When lower levels of fibrinogen are evidenced there appears to be little association between LDL and heart disease; however when higher levels of fibrinogen were noted there also appeared a greater degree of atherosclerosis.*

This adds credence to the notion that the two are partners in their combined affect on coronary heart disease. *Dr. A. Pearson, M.D., Ph.D,* responding to the question; *Should Fibrinogen levels be part of a Cardiac-Risk Workup?* answered in the affirmative. *"Yes, we measure fibrinogen levels in selected patients."*

## "The epidemiological evidence linking fibrinogen levels to later coronary events is strong, MAY BE EVEN STRONGER THAN CHOLESTEROL"

This was contained in a 1996 report. He went on to say, "fibrinogen is the best example of a new series of risk factors for thrombosis that have altered our thinking on risk factors. **No longer can we just look at stenosis.** We also have to look at *thrombogenic* factors in the blood that cause a clot to form and occlude an artery." If other study findings are correct—that *one in five might carry a defective gene for fibrinogen*—then it would follow that a genetic process would have started much earlier. Of four patients whose doctors agreed with the suggestion to test for fibrinogen, three measured scores in excess of 400 (the actual scores were 416, 420, and 461. Two of the four individuals had already <u>experienced actual first heart attacks).</u> According to data we have already looked at, those in the range of 385 or higher were in the 85% heart attack risk category.

Incidentally, it was the author's score that was the one recorded at 461. The question was, what increased risk ratio would the additional 76 points above the 385 ceiling actually add? There was no known specific medication available to lower fibrinogen, however, my score is now 260. This represents a total final reduction of approximately 45%. Most importantly, the "at-risk" component in this particular marker was diminished significantly.

# AN EARLY WARNING
# OF RISK

A 1986 fibrinogen trial performed in England produced the following remarkable results:

> **Those subjects whose scores tabulated in the *top one third* of the "normal" 200-400 reference range had an increased risk of cardiovascular disease by a measure of 84% over those study participants in the lower one third.**

Many study results are being included and referenced in this chapter because making the case against fibrinogen requires that the extended research and study results be presented to bring attention and respect to this overlooked marker in identifying another of the *"Hidden Causes of Heart Attack and Stroke."* A patient with other risk factors including claudication might benefit from being tested. In stark contrast to what has been known about *fibrinogen* is newer information supporting the theory that **plasma fibrinogen, <u>besides being an acute phase reactant</u>, is also involved with the metabolic syndrome.** One such study that came to this conclusion was conducted at the *Federico II University* in Naples, Italy. The study concluded that *hyperfibringenemia* **may be considered a component of the** *metabolic syndrome.* This would appear to further contradict the standing opinion that fibrinogen is strictly an acute phase reactant.

> **The study also confirmed: the *higher the levels of fibrinogen, the greater the health risk.***

In still another study done in Sweden, the conclusion was that plasma fibrinogen is an independent predictor of coronary heart disease and premature death in middle-aged men and even in non-smokers. We have already seen that fibrinogen among smokers promotes an even greater risk, as more and more trials indicate a direct association between this risk factor and premature death.

## WOMEN'S RISK WITH HIGH FIBRINOGEN

Although fibrinogen has been tagged as a cardiovascular risk factor for men to be concerned with, a new study has made clear the risk to the opposite sex. This Swedish study remains actually the first to have studied and calculated the risks of *cardiovascular disease and fibrinogen among women*. One can find this study in the January 1999 issue of *Arteriosclerosis, Thrombosis, and Vascular Biology*, and it is the study that was completed at the *Karolinska Institute and Hospital* in Stockholm. According to the results, the research team reported heart attacks and angina *six times higher* among women with high fibrinogen as compared to those without cardiovascular disease. Two hundred ninety two women were involved in the three-year study. The researchers in their evaluations had made adjustments for other possible contributing factors such as diabetes and smoking, previously known elements that also contribute independently to heart disease risk. *Even after these risk factors were accounted for, those women were still proven to have a **three time greater risk of heart disease!*** Another significant finding from the Swedish study was that *young women* with these factors may face an even higher risk if they also have elevated fibrinogen.

Consider that according to the information, those *premenopausal* women with the highest fibrinogen scores had a 7-FOLD INCREASED RISK compared to *postmenopausal* women.

You might recall earlier reference to smoking as an *independent contributor to increased fibrinogen levels.*

## WILL MY STATIN DRUG LOWER FIBRINOGEN?

Simvastatin (Zocor) and Lovastatin studies did not show an ability of either drug to reduce plasma fibrinogen. It would appear from the combined evidence that fibrinogen testing, at an approximate cost of $45-$55, needs to be included in the diagnostics of heart disease patients. In April of 1999, a team of researchers under the leadership of *Dr. Jing Ma* of Boston's *Channing Laboratory* compared the fibrinogen levels of 199 subjects who had experienced heart attacks during the study period with 199 subjects who did not have heart attacks.

The researchers concluded that patients in the study who had experienced heart attacks had significantly higher fibrinogen levels.

## STRESS

Haven't we been told by the medical community for as long as we can remember that smoking is bad for us? Haven't we also been told to avoid stress? Has anyone ever sat us down and explained in detail what happens to the body in response to stress? We have always been told stress hinders blood flow in the arteries, increases blood pressure. It also causes the release of harmful toxins. The Whitehall II study has now identified *fibrinogen* level increase as a new component directly responding to stress.

## FIBRINOGEN A STRESS PROTEIN
### *How your work affects your health*

The issue of stress and how it takes its toll on the body has been speculated upon for hundreds of years. There have been instances in which extreme stress has caused an individual to actually suddenly die as a consequence of overwhelming stress or intense fear. Haven't we all used the phrase "scared to death?" There have also been documented accounts where it was believed someone had literally been scared to death and rare situations (true or false) where it was speculated that someone had died in their sleep in response to an all too vivid, realistic, frightening dream. Dr. Dean Ornish, in one of his excellent books *Stress, Diet & Your Heart*, referred to a Biblical account of the man named *Ananias* who was confronted and admonished by the Apostle Peter. "You have not lied to man Ananias, you have lied to GOD!" According to the Testament account, Ananias, under grave stress, simply and inexplicably dropped dead. Here is an excellent example of "a God fearing man!" Dr. Ornish cites several other cases from history that illustrate a correlation between stress and mortality. Hospital administrators in any major city can tell you that during a natural emergency such as an earthquake or tornado some people die as a direct result of the fear and anxiety they experience. In all fairness, certain of these individuals may have already had heart rhythm disturbances, but their ultimate death was brought about by overwhelming anxiety and fear. Studies have confirmed an increase in cardiovascular related events and especially those of arrhythmic origin following 9/11. Extreme fear and stress trigger responses of both a metabolic and physiological nature, as the body releases hormones known as *catecholamines* and other toxins into the bloodstream. We all know that if we were faced with the need to run for our lives, the adrenal glands would offer up an immediate additional supply of adrenalin enabling us to run faster and longer than we could have run under normal stimuli. This short-term rush of adrenalin is a natural protective response that is well handled by the body in such emergency situations. **It is when these stress hormones and toxins are released into the blood on a repeated basis in response to stress or, for that matter, anger, a toll is taken on one's health**. Admittedly, the preceding examples were of extreme conditions, but they should serve to demonstrate how the effects of stress can contribute to illness.

## HE'S WORKING HIMSELF TO DEATH!

Ever heard that phrase before? We all have, and these age-old anecdotes are rooted somewhere in truth. *The apple doesn't fall far from the tree, still waters run deep,* and this one describing over-work and sleep deprivation, *working oneself to death.* Earlier studies have examined the phenomenon of premature death among seemingly healthy young individuals as a direct result of over-work or from extreme lack of sleep. Researchers in the Japanese *Fukuoka Heart Study* determined that among men working more than 61 hours weekly there was twice the risk of having a heart attack compared to men in the study who had been working a normal 40-hour week. The study published in volume 59 of *Occupational and Environmental Medicine* found workers **sleeping five or less hours a night raised their heart attack risk almost 3 fold.** According to this and earlier studies, sleep deprivation and "workaholic" tendencies can literally work you to an early grave!

## SOCIOECOMONIC INFLUENCES ON FIBRINOGEN

Fibrinogen has been identified as an acute phase reactant, a metabolic co-factor with type 2 diabetes, a genetically associated risk factor, and now most recently a "stress protein." How then in this recently defined role, is fibrinogen destructively involved once again? The *Whitehall II* British Government Study, determined that fibrinogen was elevated among civil service personnel in low servitude employment. The study also found a correlation between those workers who have higher levels of fibrinogen, among those who do the most work but *receive the smallest reward or recognition.* The landmark study also found chronically elevated fibrinogen levels among workers whose work is subject to the constant scrutiny and approval of others, as opposed to study subjects who make their own decisions and sail their own ship. The message one could see in these findings is that if you despise your working relationship, or the nature of your work, or are unhappy associating with those you work for, elevations in fibrinogen may be the end result. Sound incredible? In general, even people of better economic and social standing were shown to have lower stress-affected fibrinogen levels when compared to those of less social standing. Even though this study was done in the workforce, one could think of a dozen stressful situations that might just as well have been used as the criteria for a stress/fibrinogen study other than the workplace. Situations comparable to the workplace pecking order include, for example, living with an overly-critical individual who constantly berates or belittles everyone around them. There is more.

## NATURAL AND DRUG THERAPY

Several drugs have had demonstrated success in *short-term* reduction of high fibrinogen levels in critical-care situations, usually in a hospital setting and administered by injection. Included among the fibrinolytic agents are streptokinase, urokinase and tissue plasminogen activator. **Each of these drugs are administered temporarily and only under close medical supervision.** I offered a word of caution earlier, but it is now more specific to our discussion and worth repeating. Gemfibrozil, the popular *fibrate* drug, often prescribed as an excellent treatment for lowering triglycerides and for HDL increase, may also independently *raise fibrinogen levels as much as 20%*. It would seem prudent (based on this information) for patients to be monitored for fibrinogen levels while taking certain drugs with an eye on determining if they are already on the high end of the fibrinogen scale. *This is especially true for* those with an already **elevated LDL** cholesterol marker. *We spoke of a recent study that showed women with elevated fibrinogen and LDL levels as having a seven-fold increased risk of heart attack!*

# INFECTIONS AND HIGH FIBRINOGEN
## (A DANGEROUS COMBINATION)

We have been talking about evaluating the entire range of a patient's risk factors; the following entry supports that approach. An article published in the August 1999 journal *Circulation* indicated that treating infection would reduce fibrinogen levels in heart disease patients. **There is something revolutionary in this information that might affect the way doctors look at the risks of C-reactive protein, high fibrinogen and other factors that affect and contribute to heart disease.** This is certainly one of the first such breakthrough studies that confirms at least one actual path of heart disease complicated by high fibrinogen. It has long been known that fibrinogen does elevate as a result of ongoing infection. Recent studies (as we have seen) have named at least two inflammatory infections as contributors to heart disease: helicobacter pylori and chlamydia pneumoniae. As is discussed in the chapter on infections, and at the risk of repetition, an individual may unsuspectingly have had the bacteria since early childhood, unaware that he or she might have been re-infected or may have an appreciable degree of the bacterium lying dormant but inflaming the arterial walls. This recent study goes further in not only substantiating that fibrinogen is a risk factor, but also naming two particular infections whose synergistic affects might actually responsively cause elevations in fibrinogen levels and may complicate one's heart disease for years.

# CORROBORATIVE EVIDENCE
## FROM THE JOURNAL *FIBRINOLYSIS*

"Fibrinogen Level as a predictor of mortality in survivors of myocardial infarction" was reported by *Cooper J.; Douglas A.S. from the Department of Medicine and Therapeutics, Medical School, Aberdeen UK.* The levels of fibrinogen, plasminogen and activator activity were measured among seventy patients who had 4-5 years previously experienced a myocardial infarction (heart attack). At the time of these tests their coronary disease was considered stable. An independent correlation between the fibrinogen level and subsequent mortality within the following 5 years was found, over and above age and smoking. **There was a 69% increase in the risk of death associated** *with a one standard deviation increase in fibrinogen.* Among smokers, an increase of one standard deviation in fibrinogen more than doubled risk, elevating it by 2.86 times. *The message:* Heart attack victims need to monitor their fibrinogen levels and eliminate smoking to reduce their risk of another MI and to sustain a longer life. The trial results have been coming in for years and still fibrinogen and its role in cardiovascular diagnostics remains for the most part ignored. *Will the public have to wait another 29 years as they did before the homocysteine issue became accepted? Should fibrinogen be included as a marker to be evaluated along with cholesterol and other inflammatory factors?* M.D., Ph.D Edzard Ernst in 1993 concluded that *"fibrinogen can be considered a major cardiovascular risk factor."* You're a thinking person. Based on what you have read, what is your opinion? We are simply talking about identification. What is the price of not knowing when simple intervention and modification might lessen the threat? What intelligent case could be made for not testing? It may be that there hasn't been a therapy that can normalize an elevated score.

## SEARCH FOR THE REMEDY

Obviously I had a personal interest in finding a drug that could help reduce a lethal 461 fibrinogen level. The search took more than three years, until a combination of drug and natural supplements was found to successfully reduce the score some 200 points from a 461 baseline reading to a 260 endpoint. An article on fibrinogen management appearing in the journal *Atherosclerosis* had claimed that while study patients had not shown appreciable change in fibrinogen level with intake of 1,000 mgs of vitamin C, they did find increased benefit after upping the dosage to 2000 mgs. According to the study the increased intake had resulted in a favorable response in the platelet aggregation index **with a 27%** *decrease* **in fibrinogen level and a 45%** *increase* **in fibrinolytic activity.** Fibrinogen does respond to inflammatory activation. In an effort to minimize this element in my own profile, I added high doses of the proteolytic enzyme *bromelain* and the herb *turmeric*. Both have been shown to be of the most effective natural anti-inflammatory agents recognized among the alternative medicine community. On top of a vitamin C increase to 2,000 mgs was the daily intake of 7 grams of daily *omega 3 fish oil* (capsules). The remainder of the regimen included *L-arginine, green tea, cayenne pepper* (capsules), *ordorless garlic* and *niacin*. My fibrinogen dropped from the 461 level to 377, which according to the evidence was still 77 points dangerously high, and another 40 points from optimum. Now, enter into the marketplace *fenofibrate*, a new fibrate drug (at the time) for lowering triglycerides and raising

HDL. As I mentioned earlier, there has never been a drug specifically created to counter this marker. **I found in researching many drugs that the fibrate drug, *Tricor* (fenofibrate), had independently shown a side-benefit in trial of also lowering fibrinogen. It would be the only long-term drug in America that could help bring this killer into compliance.** *Bezafibrate* **is another fibrate drug, currently only available in Europe, that had also shown an ability to lower fibrinogen.**

A study published in the journal *Thrombosis and Haemostasis* 70 (2), pages 241-243, (1995) authored by Adriana Branchi and team had found that while the two popular drugs *Gemfibrozil* and *Lipitor* actually **raised** fibrinogen 20% after four months of use, *Tricor* had reduced fibrinogen by 16% (in comparison, a 36% overall difference). Not only had this new fibrate drug been proven very effective in doing what it was originally designed to do (lowering triglycerides 25% and raising HDL 23%) the drug also acted simultaneously like a statin drug, lowering total cholesterol 21%. Most important and most exciting from my point of view were the trial results that showed *Tricor* to be the only drug in America that had actually been proven to lower fibrinogen! While *simvastatin,* the statin drug in the Branchi trial, did not decrease fibrinogen, *pravastatin* did show a very minor but *inconsequential* benefit in the Italian study. Note: a second independent study published in ATVB by Marais, D.A. in 1997: 17 (8) explained the results of findings, which indicated a significant increase in fibrinogen levels among patients using *atorvastatin* (Lipitor). As outstanding a drug as Lipitor has proven to be (and it is certainly among the top statin drugs) a second independent study had actually found *increased* fibrinogen levels by more than 20% with administration of 40 BID dosage! As a safety issue, should a patient's fibrinogen level be monitored if a patient is on either of the two drugs identified as having an ability to raise fibrinogen? In my personal experience, after taking *Lipitor* for two months the fibrinogen increased *exactly* 20% and dropped when the drug was discontinued. Weight loss, cessation of smoking, aerobic exercise and running have proved beneficial in lowering this marker to some degree. Small amounts of weight reduction will not greatly reduce fibrinogen; it is a large amount of weight loss that produces the benefit. Obese individuals would be wise to have their fibrinogen levels monitored. Recent studies released from *Harvard* have found higher levels of C-reactive protein (CRP) among obese patients. CRP and fibrinogen both increase in response to inflammatory factors and weight. Almost four decades after the landmark *Framingham Heart Study* waved a red flag regarding fibrinogen's role in heart disease and stroke, the information is finally beginning to receive attention.

## SUMMARY

Atherosclerosis, in its process, builds atherosclerotic plaque. Fibrinogen is involved as a contributor if not a facilitator of this heart disease dysfunction. Elevated fibrinogen when combined with additional clotting or platelet aggregation disorders and/or with other contributing factors such as high LDL becomes even more a critical concern. High levels of fibrinogen become involved in triggering a negative cascade of thrombotic controls leading to stroke. Fibrinogen definitely qualifies as a major *Hidden Cause of Heart Attacks and Stroke*. **We will no doubt be hearing more information about this serious risk factor. It**

**may take a few years but this marker will one day be issued newer, less-forgiving guidelines and hopefully more attention paid to testing patients to learn who is actually at risk.**

We have acknowledged certain benefits of the drug fenofibrate—however, near the completion of the writing I became aware of an important conflicting study from Magdeburg, Germany. Caution: It was learned from the Jetta Dierkes study that homocysteine levels among fenofibrate users increased 40%. Monitoring homocysteine levels would be prudent.

*Someone asked recently what I thought was the most important information I had garnered from the 5 years of research. In response I explained that even though all we have discussed is important, I would have to list in no specific order the following six as outstanding vitally important breakthroughs.*

    ▶  *CRP*
    ▶  *omega 3, found in fish oil*
    ▶  *vulnerable plaque*
    ▶  *nitric oxide*
    ▶  *fibrinogen*
    ▶  *homocysteine*

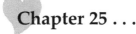

# Chapter 25

# Sounds Fishy:
# *Omega-3*

A restaurant in Los Angeles, California, formerly called the *Seafood Broiler*, more than 22 years ago hung a large plaque in the foyer of the customer waiting area. The notice paraphrased information that German researchers had come to believe that eating fish once or twice a week could substantially reduce the risk of heart disease. Those claims have been clinically substantiated to a much greater degree over these past 22 years. Here in mass for the reader's benefit, is the up-to-date overwhelming proof of benefit derived from omega 3 fish oil.

Fish oil, a source of necessary omega 3 fatty acids, provides numerous benefits not only for heart disease patients in general but for those with specific rhythmic heart disorders as well. New information indicates that it provides additional health advantage for other organs and ailments including rheumatoid arthritis and bipolar disease. **A study with 44 participants showed such remarkable results that the study was canceled prematurely in order that all**

**of the patients in the study could benefit from adding the oil to their collective diets.** The benefits to those ingesting the fish oil must have been overwhelmingly convincing to cause the premature conclusion and cancellation of an ongoing trial. Studies also suggest that fish oil benefits patients with colon cancer, depression, asthma, menstrual cramps, diabetes, multiple sclerosis and rheumatoid arthritis. The arthritis advantage is due to the oil's anti-inflammatory attributes. This particular study provided even more support for the recent information regarding the dangers of higher elevations of triglycerides, and introduced the finding that **women with higher triglyceride values are at greater risk than their male counterparts.** Fish oil has proven to have great ability to lower triglycerides but it also has been shown to reduce a woman's risk of developing heart disease. Of particular interest is information that postmenopausal women can receive additional health benefit simply by ingesting fish oil. Dr. Ken D. Stark from the *University of Guelph* in Ontario, Canada authored a study that monitored 35 postmenopausal women between ages 43-60 who had shown no history of heart disease. **Those treated with the rich omega 3 oil had 25% less risk of developing heart disease than those on placebo. The author Dr. Stark suggested that this benefit would not have been acquired just by diet alone.** The amount of intake from diet would not have been sufficient without actually including a fish oil supplement. The study can be found in the *American Journal of Clinical Nutrition*, August 2000. Fish oil supplements fall into the polyunsaturated fat category. Omega-3 is found predominately in fatty fish: trout, white tuna, halibut, salmon and mackerel. Many people who are not fish eaters per se may better handle eating canned tuna. Other seafoods high in omega-3 are oysters, sardines and herring. **Consuming any of these fatty fish can significantly re-**

**duce triglycerides.** Now that the information is on the record that levels of triglycerides over 100 are suspect, a diet adding even modest amounts of fish makes more sense than ever.

## TAKE THESE STATISTICS TO HEART

When the evidence is reviewed in its entirety, it becomes clear that omega 3's role could be absolutely lifesaving. If you took only the results of this next study to heart you would be far ahead of the game. A study reported in the *Journal of American Medical Association* followed some 20,000 men for more than 11 years. We would probably agree this is a lengthy and sizeable study from which to draw conclusion.

> **THOSE STUDY SUBJECTS WHO SAID THEY ATE FISH ONE OR MORE TIMES A WEEK HAD A 50% REDUCED RISK OF SUDDEN DEATH FROM A HEART ATTACK OVER THE FOLLOWING 10-YEAR PERIOD!**

This was in comparison to the men who only ate fish once a month.

## DEPRESSION, BIPOLAR DISEASE AND OMEGA 3

Depression, whether manifested as clinical depression or depression associated with bipolar disease, is a major national health concern. Studies have found that improvement in the symptoms of bipolar patients improved considerably while consuming a fish diet.

# FISH OIL AND LOWERED INCIDENCE OF SUDDEN DEATH

Would fish oil have prevented a good percentage of the approximately quarter million deaths of men and women yearly from sudden cardiac death and associated rhythmic heart disorders? The statistics and documented autopsy results concluded that **those persons who frequently ate fish succumbed to** *sudden death* **in much fewer numbers** than those who did not. <u>**This is not surprising, considering that when the arteries of these cadavers were examined they were found to be free from atherosclerosis!**</u>

# FISH EATERS REDUCE THEIR POST-HEART ATTACK RISK OF SUDDEN DEATH BY 29%

The prominent British peer publication *Lancet* printed the results of a two-year study of men who had previously suffered a heart attack. These men were given one of two different dietary regimens. One group was instructed to add more fiber to their diet, while the other group was asked to include one or two helpings of a fatty fish per week. *Not every day, but just two helpings over the entire week.* The results reported after two years were amazing. *The "fishy" group had experienced 29% fewer deaths* than the "fiber" group.

## UPDATE! A NEW STUDY RELEASED FOUND A DECREASE IN SUDDEN DEATH BY 81%!

In the *New England Journal of Medicine*'s April/2002 edition, the results of the *Physicians Health Study* on the benefit of eating fish a few times per week were announced. From the 22,000 doctors whose evaluation had begun 20 years earlier, the following result was recorded:

> **Men in the study without any known heart attack risks were 81% less likely to die of a heart attack and sudden death than those who did not eat fish.**

What might account for the large difference between 29% and 81%? The earlier study had required fish once or twice a week whereas the later *Physician's Study* reported the participants having fish several times a week.

Almost simultaneously, a 16-year *Harvard School of Public Health* study also supported the findings of the *Physician Health Study*, determining that among 80,000 nurses surveyed, a decreased risk of developing heart disease or actually dying from heart attack was attributed to the polyunsaturated fat from omega 3 fish oil.

## GOOD NEWS FOR STROKE RISK

As exciting as this information might be for heart attack survivors, there were even more dramatically favorable results in a Dutch trial involving some 552 men. Here the study did not concentrate on heart disease but rather on **stroke,** *the other killer* we are concerned with. Outstandingly the study reported a whopping *51% reduction from the normally expected stroke statistics.* **A 51% reduction in stroke is quite simply a major accomplishment!**

# PROOF POSITIVE
*For those who have already experienced an MI*

*Lancet* introduced the results of the work of Dr. Roberto Marchioli of Santa Maria Imbaro, Italy. In actuality, this particular study was implemented to study the difference between vitamin E benefit compared to that of fish oil among post MI (heart attack) cases. This three and half year study had been formulated to rule in or rule out earlier studies that claimed vitamin E (if taken after a heart attack) would reduce future cardiovascular events.

# THE STUDY RESULTS

This Italian study involving 11,000 heart patients reported that the n-3 fatty acids found in fish and fish oil significantly decreased the rate of death by lessening the number of fatal heart attacks and stroke. Taking fish oil supplements resulted in a reduced risk of dying from fatal or nonfatal heart attack or stroke compared to patients who did not take the supplements. The incidence of SUDDEN DEATH could be significantly reduced simply by adding a weekly meal of "fatty" fish. The indications certainly are that consuming fish reduces the risk of experiencing a deadly heart attack. There are, of course, two kinds.

## SUMMARY

You've been presented the results of millions of patient study hours gathered from numerous studies. The collective results strongly list in the favorable column, regular intake of omega 3 from fish oil for the treatment and prevention of cardiovascular disease and stroke.

# Chapter 26

# COMBINATION
# *Therapy*

What is it? Can it really provide benefit for those patients with stubborn lipid profiles? Combination therapy, a relatively new approach to the management of difficult lipid profiles, is gaining more and more popularity among leading-edge physicians and cardiologists. The *National Cholesterol Education Program* has suggested a more aggressive approach to help complex lipid disorder patients achieve the recommended levels. It is known that many cholesterol-lowering drugs have the capability of reducing LDL levels some 30% or more. However, in the theoretical case of a patient who presents a mean LDL cholesterol of say 210, and after much honest sacrifice and effort only succeeds in bringing the level down to 147 (30% lower), that level would still be considered an unacceptably high LDL level. Often individuals with very high cholesterol (265-280 or even higher) find that they and their doctors become frustrated over the lack of success in gaining control of these adverse lipid profiles, even though rigorous dietary, exercise and traditional drug therapies have already been employed. Perhaps you know someone who has felt that same frustration. The situation is not unlike that of a person who has tried every diet without success, while someone else using the very same diet loses weight and ends up looking like their high school graduation picture. What else is available in the arsenal when after dedicated effort one fails to reach the desired endpoints? Where should the patient and doctor turn? What other means of control may be implemented? Several trials responding to these very questions have shown remarkable results. As with any medicinal approach there can be complications, and physicians weigh the risks for and against the use of combination therapy.

Combination therapy will prove to be a most viable strategy for treating these difficult cases. A study done at the *Hadassah University Hospital, Jerusalem, Israel* which appeared in the *American Journal of Cardiology* July 7, 1995 focused on this very problem. The reporting team had studied the safety of *triple therapy* using statin, fibrate, and resin drugs all at the same time. The combination of the different type drugs produced a 40.4%-52.5% reduction of cholesterol levels during the sixty-day study. There have been other multiple drug studies using different combinations that have posted very significant results as well. Combination therapy is used effectively in treating many other diseases, including cancer, and HIV where patients have benefited from three drugs administered in the "drug cocktail." Combinations have been effective in prolonging life in many cases. A combination remedy is not without substance and is not a unique approach. Immediate questions come to mind concerning the wisdom and efficacy of adding additional medications to one's current therapy. An obvious first question might be, why not simply double or triple the dosage of what the patient is currently taking?

# DON'T RAISE THE WATER, LOWER THE BRIDGE!

Trials exploring doubling or tripling dosage in a monolithic one-drug approach in difficult profiles have returned results that have not been all that encouraging. Too often in these complex lipid disorder cases this approach has met with diminishing returns. For example, the single drug one is currently assigned may be attacking cholesterol adequately in <u>one specific manner</u>. It may produce a very positive effect for instance on the LDL, but the HDL may not be responding as effectively as hoped for when the regimen had begun. Also, a statin drug may be dealing very well with the LDL/HDL ratio, but in some patients with multiple lipid disorder, the same drug may not be delivering the required and anticipated response in controlling triglycerides, particularly in favorably adjusting the tryglyceride/HDL ratio. While one drug is attacking the cholesterol from one direction, another drug added to the program by the physician might attack cholesterol from a quite different direction. The combination in this individualized therapeutic prescription may be just what the doctor ordered for very difficult lipid cases, or at least based on the evidence, should order.

# YOU CAN'T WIN A WAR JUST WITH AIR SUPPORT!

They talk in the news of not being able to win any battle overseas with just air support. Military strategists drawing their battle plans will determine that a combination approach by land, air and sea are required to accomplish the objective. In dealing with cholesterol the combination battle group might include statin drugs which attack the enemy *at the liver*, a sequestrant bile acid drug whose approach is to attack the digestive supply lines *in the stomach*, and perhaps yet another ally from the vitamin attack squadron, the B vitamin niacin, (nicotinic acid), which is itself a drug and should be treated with the same respect. The war has already begun and a strategy of combination lipid therapy may accomplish the desired effect where single drug administration has previously failed. Whether or not you enlist in this particular battle is a decision to be weighed between you and your physician.

## MULTIPLE DRUG THERAPY RESULTS

In one representative study, patients were placed on either placebo or drug therapy and instructed in a normal lipid lowering diet. Participants were entered into the program based on having shown a 30% stenosis (blockage) of one major artery and elevated total cholesterol. They were randomly assigned to "blinded drug therapy" or matching placebo (no one knew if they were on placebo or an actual drug). Treatment was begun singularly, with pravastatin (*Pravachol*), nicotinic acid (B vitamin), cholestyramine (a bile acid drug) and Gemfibrozil (a fibrate drug). Each would be added individually to the program at intervals between 6-12 weeks as the trial progressed, until the desired lipid (cholesterol) levels were attained. Once the study clinicians and doctors reached the desired endpoints, they monitored the subjects continually every three months for the next 2.5 years. Patient safety was, as always, of major primary importance.

# THE STUDY RESULTS

**93% of those in the treatment group reached the target lipid levels!** A pretty dramatic success rate.

Apparently, there may be hope in combination therapy for those who have been discouraged by all their prior attempts to reach desired lipid levels.

It took an average of approximately six months (23 weeks) to achieve these desired affects. In the first phase in which Pravastatin (Pravachol) was the only drug introduced, LDL cholesterol alone was reduced by an impressive 32% percent. It is worth noting that with this 32% reduction most people with elevated LDL levels would probably fall into the desired range of acceptable LDL levels. However, the trial findings were most impressive for those complex profiles that even after the 32% reduction still remained at a significant high point of risk. Enter now **phase two,** and addition of nicotinic acid (niacin) into the program between 6-12 weeks. *Niacin* brought the test subject's LDL down an additional 11% in 40 out of 44 cases. When the third drug, *cholestyramine,* was introduced, a negative response was noted. This drug actually raised triglyceride levels and lowered, undesirably, the HDL level. *Gemfibrozil,* when added as the fourth drug, accomplished nothing. *In the final analysis, the two drugs Pravachol and nicotinic acid (Niacin) were effective in reaching the desired levels in patients whose therapy had previously been ineffective.* There were similar results obtained in another study using Simvastatin (*Zocor*) and niacin. There is a point of diminishing returns in the currently accepted approach, when doubling or tripling the dosage in mono-lithic one drug therapy would probably not attain these same outstanding results. Cholesterol readings, including both total and LDL cholesterol, continued to rise in the *placebo* group during the course of the trial. Conversely, those on the drug therapy continued to enjoy lowered LDL lipid panels. Among those assigned combination therapy, HDL (good cholesterol) rose a significant average amount of 25%.

## REGRESSION: REALITY OR PIE IN THE SKY?

Is regression a reality? Can artery disease actually be reversed? If so, show me! What is the evidence? The public has been trying to get its mind around just controlling cholesterol and now there is talk of actual regression. It has been established in certain combination regression studies like the one just discussed that different approaches, in combination, may bring a new dimension to the battle.

## REGRESSION PROBABLILITY

Regression is the desirable goal and according to the results of several trials, leading cardiologists believe that it is attainable.

*" In general, the results to date in humans and experimental animals seem to indicate that substantial regression of advanced atherosclerosis is possible. "*

**—Wissler RW, Vesslinovitch**

The results also indicate that advanced atherosclerotic lesions are much more likely to respond favorably if LDL serum cholesterol concentrations are reduced to the minimum. This next entry should be encouraging to anyone on cholesterol drugs. According to Vesslinovitch, you can truly reverse the condition.

*"This value* **(for reversal)** *appears to be about 150 mg and under these circumstances, much of the lipid disappears from the plaques...calcium can be removed from the advanced plaques and consistently produce regression of advanced atherosclerotic lesions in human subjects."*

Isn't that good news?

You might recall in an earlier chapter William Castelli's findings following the *Framingham* indicated that none of 5,000 patients with cholesterol readings of 150 or lower died of heart disease or suffered a heart attack in the 25 years since the actual trial. The *Harvard Atherosclerosis Reversibility Project Study Group* has been involved in at least one trial to monitor and determine the efficacy and tolerability of such multi-drug therapy. Superko and Krauss assessing the viability of this particular regressive therapy and after analyzing the results of several regressive studies, published their conclusions in journal *Circulation* August of 1994. The article was entitled **Coronary Artery Disease Regression; Convincing evidence for the benefit of aggressive lipoprotein management.** Reporting on ten randomized, controlled clinical trials, the two doctors found that the evidence more than suggested, coronary artery disease indeed could be arrested by the management of our lipids. When the final results were in which included a large number of 2,095 subjects from ten separate studies, the results of the therapeutic approach of combination therapy was found to be very significant.

# Chapter 27

# *Aneurysms*

An aneurysm, non-medically speaking, may be described as a bulge in an artery, not unlike a large area that might appear in a bicycle or automobile tire. Blow too much air into a balloon and it can produce what is often referred to as a "goose egg."

Uncontrolled blood pressure can produce the same results with a weakened arterial wall and the "blowing out" of the wall's structure. In this condition, an aneurysm (depending on its size), is vulnerable to burst or rupture at any time. The final result of such a catastrophic event usually results in death.

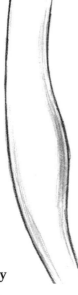

**Fig 8(a): Bulging artery**

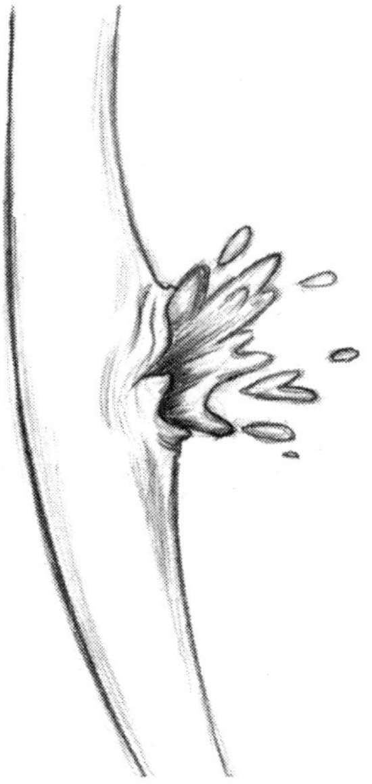

Fig 8(b): Bursting artery

A patient would have to be in a controlled setting in a medical facility to have any chance at all. Even then the chances would be nebulous at best. The national statistics endorse the fact that some 15,000 lives a year are lost to this type of rupture where the aorta joins at the stomach. This rupture is called an *abdominal aortic aneurysm* (AAA). There are other sites for aneurysm including the brain and the actual heart or aorta itself. The strongest chance a patient has comes with early detection.

Aneurysms are very often caused by advanced atherosclerosis as a build-up of fatty plaques weaken the artery wall. It is here where the process of hemorrhage and repair is repeated time and again.

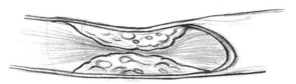

Fig 9: Plaque build-up on artery wall

The second complication is called *turbulence,* a condition that is created by the pressure of blood flow as it pounds and erodes against the bends and turns of a plaque-narrowed artery. Over time the cumulative attacks weaken the artery's integrity and an aneurysm forms.

## ANEURYSMS ARE OFTEN INHERITED AND DO RUN IN FAMILIES

If you find aneurysm in your investigation of family history, the doctor would be most interested in hearing about it. There are different non-invasive procedures to locate aneurysms, one is a doppler ultrasound. "Watchful waiting" is considered the proper standard of care in cases where (according to the guidelines) an aneurysm has not met the critical criteria. There is a window of surgical opportunity that is determined by the actual size of the aneurysm. In most cases when the diseased section increases to the designated size, the decision is made to operate.

## A CASE HISTORY OF INHERITANCE

A golf pro I knew attended his twin brother's funeral in Phoenix, Arizona several years ago. The deceased brother's doctor, also a friend, attended the ceremony. Not surprisingly, he was struck by the physical similarity of the twin brother, who was serving as one of the pallbearers. The doctor approached my friend after the burial and asked him when he was planning on leaving Phoenix. The brother was scheduled to return to Los Angeles the following morning. The doctor convinced the brother to come to his office before he left for a quick examination at no charge. The doctor discovered a large ABDOMINAL AORTIC ANEURYSM IN EXACTLY THE SAME SPOT where the deceased twin brother had his. The doctor scheduled his new patient for immediate surgery. Although the doctor had lost one twin, his quick thinking and intervention probably saved the other. This doctor was practicing the "art" of medicine; enough said.

## COPPER AND ANEURYSM

Copper, according to certain studies, provides some prophylaxis against developing aneurysms. Anyone with atherosclerosis or a family history of aneurysms would probably benefit from adding this mineral to their regimen. From a preventive standpoint, health-minded people in general should include 2 milligrams daily. Multiple vitamins usually will have this amount. In the case of copper, **more is not better**; 2 mgs is the recommended dosage.

A new procedure has just been given the approval of the FDA for application in the treatment of AAA (*abdominal aorta aneurysm*). It is a non-invasive procedure that is already available in more than 20 facilities across the country. The procedure, known as the AneuRx Stent Graft System, involves the threading of a catheter through an incision in the groin upward into the abdominal aorta to the location of the aneurysm. The procedure, not unlike the angioplasty procedure, involves the insertion and permanent placement of a *sleeve stent.* The stent serves to relieve the pressure on the aneurysm. The procedure is reportedly enjoying a 92% success rate. The FDA has approved two devices, the *Ancure Tube and Bifurcated Endovascular Grafting System* and the *AneuRx Stent Graft System.*

# Chapter 28

# - SMOKING -

## *a controllable* **Risk Factor**

Here is a particular controllable independent risk factor that must be eliminated from one's lifestyle. It seems more and more young people in spite of the warnings are joining the ranks of smokers. Since I am attempting to address the many causes of heart disease, both those that are inherited and those with environmental or behavioral links, I would be remiss to not include the modifiable health threat of smoking. **After all, it has the dubious distinction of being at the very top of the list of heart attack risk factors. Numero uno!**

## SMOKING STILL THE
## NUMBER ONE RISK FACTOR

According to the Pan American Health Organization (PAHO), 625,000 Americans die every year from tobacco use. It is no longer debatable. You may be aware of the landmark superior court decision ruling that held the tobacco companies culpable and liable for reimbursing the state's treasuries to the tune of some 206 billion dollars for the costs of illness and death resulting from chronic smoking. All the while the tobacco companies had maintained that *they were not convinced that nicotine was addictive.* The court based its opinion on expert witness testimony that proved otherwise. Not only had tobacco company executives known of tobacco's addictive properties, they had actually ordered research to ensure and enhance their product's addictive properties. For the sake of preventive healthcare and certainly for the prevention of heart disease, doctors and the medical profession at large are obligated to educate people properly and to disseminate information on this highly addictive drug. A doctor will tell you that high blood pressure is a cardiovascular risk and recognize the importance of its control. They will also attack high cholesterol, but when it comes to smoking, **THE NUMBER ONE RISK FACTOR** (according to national studies), doctors have failed in convincing their at-risk patients to stop. In one study the rate of cardiovascular events among smokers was 2.3 times greater than among non-smokers. In another study that measured the effort in most all United States medical schools, Doctor Linda Ferry, a faculty member of the *Loma Linda School of Medicine* released the following statement.

*"A majority of U.S. medical students are not adequately trained to treat nicotine dependence, the most costly and deadly preventable health problem in the United States."*

Dr. Ferry's study results were published in the *Journal of the American Medical Association*. In an article released by the *Reuters* news service, Ferry's answer to the question of why the lack of concentrated approach existed was, **"All of us who are the faculty in medical schools were never trained. We study diabetes, we study heart disease. We had to learn by the seat of our pants about HIV...we felt pressure there so we developed those skills."** Dr. Ferry went on to explain, "But there's no importance in treating tobacco, very few insurance companies will reimburse." She also said during the interview, "You get paid for ulcers, hypertension, but you don't get paid for helping someone stop smoking. The impression is you stop when you are ready with safe, over the counter drugs." She went on to say, *"doctors do not do well when it comes to behavioral problems."*

In all fairness, doctors might have warned their patients many times, but when the patient's promises to quit turn out to be empty promises, the doctors might have felt their words were falling on deaf ears. Perhaps too often mincing of words in an effort to not alienate or lose the patient may be counter-productive, while a more direct approach would make a much stronger impression. By way of contrast, consider the stance a doctor in Winnipeg Canada made in early 2002, when he informed his patients, **"if you are going to continue to smoke, get yourself a new doctor!"** Somewhere, there is a disconnect; somehow, the intellect hears the warnings, but the body does not respond. **Does this not sound like one of the symptoms of classic drug dependency?** The bottom line is, smoking is not an easy habit to quit. We have all made suggestions to friends and family members that we thought would be helpful; statistics you have just read will help someone make the point more powerfully. Overall, based on the growing number of young smokers, it would be safe to say <u>the message presented has not been a persuasive one</u>.

# WOMEN, STROKE AND THAT LETHAL CIGARETTE

It was considered glamorous in those films of the forties or fifties when Betty Davis or Lauren Bacall would take those long sensual drags on a cigarette. With the pressure brought to bear by the anti-smoking establishment, smoking on film became almost non-existent. That is, until the mid and late nineties, when more and more scenes included the ambiance of that *stinking* layer of second-hand smoke drifting across the screen and into the consciousness of the public—particularly, it seems, the consciousness of the younger public who **are acquiring the dangerous habit in alarming numbers.**

# HOW QUICKLY CAN A YOUNG PERSON BECOME ADDICTED TO SMOKING?

According to Dr. Joseph R. Diorama, *University of Massachusetts Medical Center in Worcester, "Nicotine addiction occurs much more quickly in adolescents than we thought was possible."*

Many youngsters who admitted to **smoking just once a week, showed a degree of nicotine dependence in as little as 2 weeks;** in another study with 681 adolescents, 21 in the study **showed symptoms of dependence within four weeks.**

## WOMEN SMOKERS, CONSIDER THIS

> *"The greatest single contributor to the death rate among women that can be altered and controlled, is smoking.* The most prevalent risk factor preventable, is smoking."

Incidentally, this information applies not just to cigarettes but to cigars as well. As chic as the fad has become, the *Surgeon General* would issue warnings on packages indicating that there are also serious health concerns associated with smoking cigars. Here are a few of the various captions that must appear on the labels of the products of the seven largest cigar manufacturers as a result of a suit brought against them by the *Federal Trade Commission* (FTC).

1. **"Tobacco use increases the risk of lung cancer and heart disease"**
2. **"Cigar smoking can cause cancers of the mouth and throat, even if you don't inhale"**
3. **"Tobacco use increases the risk of infertility, stillbirth and low birth weight"**
4. **"Cigars are not a safe alternative to cigarettes"**

Young women: smoking may *double your risk of heart attack even if you would call yourself an occasional smoker.* One cigarette a day, according to a team of British health investigators, increases one's chances of a heart attack. Four hundred fifty women (ages 16 to 44) were included in this British study. The participants had more in common than just being light smokers. Each already had experienced a heart attack within the previous six years. According to the findings published in the journal *Heart* in the December issue 1999, **women who just smoked between *one to five* cigarettes a day (not packs mind you) increased their heart attack risk two hundred percent.** They had twice the risk of a non-smoker. The following statistic is an alarming one.

**THOSE WOMEN IN THE STUDY WHO SMOKED TWO PACKS OF CIGARETTES A DAY WERE 75 TIMES MORE IN DANGER OF A HEART ATTACK THAN NON-SMOKING WOMEN.**

In addition there is the association of certain types of cancer and, most certainly, gum disease.

## CIGARS "ACUTE IMPAIRMENT" TO THE ARTERIES

*Women and teenagers have accounted for the 30% increase in cigar smoking in the past three years.* New evidence reported by Dr. Minerva Santo Thomas and her team of researchers claimed that cigar smoking affects the arteries differently and more immediately than cigarette smoking. **This new information pokes a hole in the theory that smoking that stylish *"stogie"* is a less harmful substitute for the cigarette. Not so, according to this clinical study which supports the notion that blood flow is immediately impaired when one smokes a cigar.** The damage is immediate to the endothelium cells that are located within the artery. The researchers suggested that the reduced dilation of the arteries among cigar smokers reduces the effectiveness of blood flow and oxygen to the body tissues. Even the heart muscle itself may be subjected to added risk during bouts of exercise and certainly times of stress when the restricted vessels are permitting even less blood flow. **A person with compromised blood flow as a result of heart disease is immediately put at unsuspected risk while believing the hype that cigars are less dangerous to one's health and an attractive alternative to cigarette smoking.**

These dangers could be presented innocently to you or me through second hand smoke from unconcerned co-workers, spouses, or friends who insist on lighting up in our presence. According to one study, postmenopausal women who have continued or *recently begun smoking* may accordingly have a higher risk of developing arterial blockages in the carotid arteries. These women who have recently joined the ranks of smokers strangely enough have the unenviable distinction of possessing an *even greater risk of suffering a stroke than those women who have smoked for a much longer time*. These claims were made in a March 11, 1997 issue of the journal *Stroke* by a Dr. P.H. Holly, C. Lassila at the *University of Pittsburgh School of Public Health.*

> **Those women who smoked had five times the risk of developing at least one fatty deposit (blockage) clinging to the vessel wall...**

as opposed to those women who have never had the inclination to emulate Betty Davis, Lauren Bacall or for that matter cigar-smoking celebrities like Demi Moore. Information claimed that those women who were just beginning to smoke in their postmenopausal status were *at higher risk of stroke than women who have never smoked.* The report was published in the *American Heart Association* journal *Stroke.* **The message is clear: if you don't smoke, don't start. If you <u>do</u> smoke, quit.**

# Chapter 29

# Diabetes and Heart Disease,
## a *Destructive Alliance*

You cannot present a book on cardiovascular disease and not include information on *diabetes mellitus* (already mentioned more than 20 times). The two chronic diseases are often joined at the hip, or perhaps more accurately at the heart.

More than 16 million Americans are affected by type 2 diabetes, a form of the disease that *contributes* to some 200,000 deaths a year in this country alone. These figures are separate from the 300,000 children with juvenile onset diabetes. In plain words, these children are going to be dealing with this very serious (and expensive) disease that might have well been controlled by diet and exercise during childhood. The disease is gaining converts at an alarming rate. Sixty-one percent of the US adult population is considered obese. The national numbers have doubled since 1980, even though the information concerning maintaining a proper diet and increasing exercise has been well publicized. Isn't it ironic that the biggest health problem in many countries is fighting off starvation, while we in America are striving to fight off overeating? As a population we are literally eating ourselves into an early grave, and spending billions of dollars on diets and excess food in the process. The complications of the two maladies, heart disease and diabetes, particularly among those patients with (type II) adult onset diabetes, provide a major challenge for both the patient and the doctor. *As if one by itself were not difficult enough to treat, the task becomes monumental when the two present themselves together in a patient's profile.*

The *American Heart Association* presented a paper entitled *Diabetes Patients Are In The Dark Concerning Heart Disease.* In May, 2001 the study report found that 63% of diabetic patients suffer from one or more cardiovascular problems, plus a significant percentage of these patients must deal with high blood pressure. There is additional information acquired from performing numerous angioplasties and open-heart surgeries documenting that 80% of patients die of blood vessel or heart disease. Diabetes is a vascular disease.

> **The report stated that adults with diabetes have two to four times the risk of suffering a heart attack or stroke than those without diabetes.**

This is a disease that can sneak up on you. Unless familial history provides a warning, most people are unaware and unconcerned of the risk until they are diagnosed. The AHA has warned that diabetic patients must aggressively monitor and control blood pressure. This concerted, intense control can lower stroke by 44% and lessen the risk of kidney and eye disease complications. Controlling cholesterol (and particularly triglycerides) is also a critical part of a diabetic's therapy, and tryglyceride/HDL ratios need careful attention. According to Sydney C. Smith, Jr., M.D., *Chief Science Officer for the American Heart Association*,

> "Research from the past few years has helped us better understand the link between diabetes and cardiovascular disease, and the role *insulin resistance* plays in both." The scientist went on to say, "The American Heart Association considers diabetes one of the other major risk factors for cardiovascular disease. Unfortunately, diabetes patients still try to treat heart disease as a separate disease."

## DIABETES AND SYNDROME X

A patient who presented with *hypertension, low HDL cholesterol, obesity and elevated triglycerides* was proven to be at much greater risk of developing diabetes. Somewhere along the way researchers labeled this combination "Syndrome X." Newest research indicates that fibrinogen as well as elevated uric acid levels increase heart attack risk among syndrome X patients.

## INSULIN RESISTANCE

Insulin resistance is a term that describes the manner in which the body sends false signals causing the pancreas to overwork. When we look to the landmark PROCAM /

MUNSTER STUDY, the findings on various cardiovascular risk factors when in conjunction with hypertension and diabetes are extremely alarming. For example when a patient's heart disease was complicated by *both hypertension and diabetes* the patient experienced an 8 times added risk of heart attack! The American Association of Endocrinologists recently spoke out collectively, identifying those in danger of developing diseases linked to obesity. The following list of warning signs was given to signal which individuals were in the danger zone and may be on their way to developing congestive heart failure, sleep apnea and or diabetes.

- **Over age 45**
- **A man's waist size exceeding 40 inches**
- **A woman's waist size exceeding 35 inches**
- **Blood pressure above 130/85**
- **"Fasting" blood sugar readings over 110.**

If you or someone you know has entered, or is at risk of entering, the risk ranges above, they need to take action to reduce their risk. Most often simply losing 10-15 lbs and regular exercise will make the difference.

Most of us are probably aware that diabetes can cause blindness in its advanced stage as tiny blood vessels within the eye rupture. If these hemorrhages are not in the central vision, laser therapy can often be administered to cauterize the ruptures. In the case of central vision hemorrhage as with patients complicated with macular degeneration, laser use would burn the optic nerve as the beam would penetrate through the center region, blinding the patient. Another major concern the doctor and diabetic patient face is the constant threat of infection that creates the necessity for an estimated 54,000 amputations of lower limbs each year. There is some good news, however, according the *Diabetes Prevention Program* (DPP) study.

---

**Diabetes is a controllable disease if risk factors are closely monitored and patients become more involved in simple health style modifications including diet and exercise.**

---

You might have seen news reports that have focused more attention on the dramatic increase of obesity among children. This increase is also obvious among the general adult population. According to released figures, there has been an increase of obesity in more than 75% of young adults. The innocent child 20 or 40 pounds overweight with the cute countenance, or the young adult who is in the same overweight category and possibly living a sedentary lifestyle, may one day needlessly become one of the 16+ million diabetic patients suffering from this serious illness. It doesn't have to be this way, not with the good news coming out of the research community that behavioral adjustment in diet and even 30 minutes of daily exercise can remove the majority of patients from this disease equation. **Yes, diabetes, according to the information, is a controllable disease**.

Obesity, pot-bellies, and a high mid-body and hip to upper body index ratio are all indications that someone is headed for a diagnosis of diabetes. Health agencies have voiced concerns over the detriment to the health of individuals and to the system as a whole as this disease spirals out of control. The *Behavioral Risk Factor Surveillance System* (BFRSS) focused national attention on the actual costs of this disease and concluded statistically that in this country the dollar amount of treating diabetes among both in and out of hospital patients, combined with a loss of productivity, disability and premature death, was in excess of 98 billion dollars! These figures had been generated from a report several years earlier. At just 30%, a complete cost adjustment increase since the earlier study, the amount today would be approximately 30 billion dollars higher.

# Chapter 30

# Physical Exertion and MI's

## EARLY MORNING HEART ATTACKS

Is there a marked increase of heart attacks in the early morning hours as opposed to other times? Apparently, judging by the results of numerous studies (including the *Framingham Heart Study*), the answer is yes. In the *Determinants of Onset of Myocardial Infarction Study*, as sponsored by the *National Institutes of Health*, 1800 patient subjects were interviewed (post heart attack) in a search to better identify and understand dangerous mechanisms that might trigger heart attacks. The following was a significant finding.

**HEAVY EXERTION WAS IDENTIFIED AS THE MECHANISM THAT PRODUCED A 5.9 TIMES HIGHER RISK OF EPISODE WITHIN ONE HOUR OF THE ACTUAL PHYSICAL EXERTION.**

There proved to be a large difference in the degree of risk between those subjects who <u>exercised many times a week</u>, and those who only performed minimally or infrequently. This distinction would fall under the general heading of "being in shape" as opposed to being the proverbial "weekend warrior." Among the sedentary individuals who exerted themselves heavily less than once per week there was a higher risk compared to a significantly lower percentage among individuals that underwent heavy exertion more than five times a week. This was reported in a November, 1991 issue of *The Journal of The American Heart Association*. This very edition also carried a report from *Hartford Hospital*, in Connecticut.

**The study by Dr. Satyendra Giri and team found the risk of heart attack to be ten times greater among those subjects who maintained very low activity and had "several" contributing risk factors.**

These risk factors are already pretty well established: overweight, smoking, male gender, elevated blood pressure and elevated cholesterol. The study compared 1,048 MI patients who had experienced a heart attack **within one hour of exercising** compared to those patients who had sustained heart attacks *without* having exercised. The risk was determined to be **ten times greater among the individuals who had not exercised within the prior one hour time period**. The modes of exercise most cited were jogging, running and heavy lifting (which corresponds with the Framingham report's earlier findings). From a purely practical standpoint, consider a person who exercised regularly who was suddenly put in a position of having to expend great physical output as in running for help or being involved in an unavoidable physical confrontation. This person would have a better chance of not experiencing a heart attack from the unexpected crisis compared to a less conditioned individual. He would also have a similar advantage in much less dramatic situations such as pushing a stalled automobile out of traffic, or hand delivering a refrigerator to a mother-in-law's new third floor apartment because his wife had generously volunteered his services. An annual treadmill on one's physical exam requires the patient to be extended to the outer limits of their endurance. For those sedentary individuals anticipating such exertion, it might be wise to embark on some kind of low-intensity conditioning even if it were simply walking in the days or weeks prior to the exercise treadmill exam.

We are looking at many of the different causes of heart attacks and stroke. There is *one* area of risk that should not be overlooked. This is one that we have actual control over in individual behavioral management. **Anger** is a risk factor to be included in the total spectrum of causes for heart attack and stroke. **Remember: the full dimension has to be dealt with if one wants to be truly effective in preventing a heart attack or stroke.**

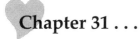

# Chapter 31

# *Anger*

In the course of writing this book, I encountered three different individuals who (along with their doctors) had not been able to explain the immediate reason for their heart attacks and (with their physician's approval) chose to explore further. The first gentleman, from New York, spoke to his physician about having blood tests run at the *Berkeley Heartlab*. The doctor and patient were both surprised at the results. This particular patient had a high *H. pylori* infection combined with a fibrinogen level of 420, along with a high reading on an inherited LP (a) gene. Perhaps most important to the discussion was the fact that the gentleman had engaged in what he described as a *severely* heated argument with a partner during a business dispute. He could not remember a time in his life when he had been more upset. *He experienced a heart attack within three hours of the incident.* Of the other individuals, (a medical professional) did not have the blood tests run, but (as we will see) did have something in common with the other two individuals. This second man shared that he too had become involved in an argument prior to his heart attack. The argument ensued during a telephone conversation with his wife. He described the distasteful encounter as the worst confrontation he had ever remembered having in his life. Apparently, he had come home from a business trip to find his wife had taken the children and moved out of the house without prior warning, leaving absolutely nothing behind except him. *Within two hours of his emotional upset, he experienced his heart attack.* The third man, whom I had known for many years, *had gotten into a violent argument at a family wedding.* He did not actually have a heart attack, but described a paralyzing agonizing pain in his lower abdomen as if something had "snapped." I convinced him to seek the evaluation of a physician, who sent him to a cardiologist who performed an echocardiogram identifying an abdominal aneurysm 5.5 centimeters in size, at risk of rupture. He was operated on in due haste. It was learned that he also had severe thoracic aortic calcification, and the aortic valve was regurgitating blood. The arotic valve was replaced with a mechanical one. Was the emotional strain of his earlier argument the added pressure on an already diseased artery that resulted in the nearly ruptured aneurysm? He believed so and still does. In casual conversation I had asked all three the same elemental question:

**" Had you lost your temper or had you been involved in an emotionally-charged hostile situation within very few hours prior to your attack? "**

## TEMPER, HOSTILITY, ANGER
## Major Risk Factors (withheld or released)

There is corroborative evidence from clinical studies that many people who have had a heart attack or stroke did so within two hours after losing their temper or reaching a high point of anxiety. Can you recall seeing movies or TV shows where a middle-aged or older man loses his temper in a dramatic scene, grabs his chest, and falls dead to the floor? It was an overused bit of business in many of the older western movies. The actor was usually seen sprawled out on the floor attempting to get to his nitroglycerin tablets, which happened to have rolled just out of reach. Often times, the disgruntled wife or business partner would simply ensure the man's fate by making sure the bottle of pills was jusssssttt unattainable. Have we been watching the same movies, you and I? How many times have we seen Spencer Tracy, Melvin Douglas or Edward G. Robinson re-enact this scenario? Well, according to the information that has come out of the cardiovascular research community regarding anger, resentment, and old fashioned hostility, these scenes were not necessarily all that exaggerated. A report published in *CARDIOLOGY TODAY* found that...

**Middle-aged men who frequently express high levels of anger and hostility have twice the stroke risk.**

A high degree of anger, already linked to development of coronary heart disease morbidity and mortality, had now been associated with an increased risk of stroke. The data was compiled from the *Kuopio Ischemic Heart Disease* study. It seems to me we have always known of the association. How many times have you heard someone advise a relative to calm down before they have a stroke? It wasn't from a scientific study but it was good common sense advice.

## WOMEN AND ANGER

Women harboring anger and hostility have a similar risk to men. A *New York Times* health article explained that each episode of anger or hostility sets off physiological responses in the body which include higher blood pressure, accelerated heart rate and narrowing of the coronary arteries. The blood actually becomes more *viscous* and literally thickens. If the person already has a high level of fibrinogen, hematocrit, or other hematologic or inflammatory complications, it is not difficult to understand how he or she might be more prone to either a heart or "brain" attack (stroke). Susan A. Everson, M.D. gave a presentation at the *70th Annual Scientific Sessions of the American Heart Association* entitled *Anger, Expression, Style, Increases Risk of Stroke in Middle-Aged Men.* The information she presented, suggested a health risk in the relationship between expression of anger, hostility and incidence of *stroke*. What made this study unique were the findings suggesting that higher levels of hostility and anger are also associated with hypertension and carotid artery disease. *For the first time a study looked at these psychological traits and their involvement in incidence of stroke and mortality.* For the record, a stroke occurs every 53 seconds in this country.

## WOMEN'S RISK WITH SUPRESSED ANGER

The final report of a 10-year study from the *University of Pittsburgh School of Medicine* was published in the 8/1998 issue of *Psychosomatic Medicine*. Middle-aged women who suppress anger, have hostile attitudes, or feel self-conscious in public, may face greater risk of developing cardiovascular disease. The study also indicated that women who continue with these feelings have a greater tendency to develop carotid artery disease. Using just a grain of common sense, one could include other contributing situations. Imagine the stress and righteous anger that builds in a woman who has been the recipient of abuse from a domineering, overbearing husband who has belittled or intimidated her, or even perpetrated physical violence upon her person, for years. Lingering anger over time can not only raise blood pressure, but can also *wreak physical damage on the heart muscle*. Whether feelings of anger are held within or are released, the overall cumulative effect appears (judging from the evidence) to remain the same. This by itself is interesting, because it has always seemed to follow that someone who loses their temper or screams his or her anger outwardly was better off for having released it. Not so, according to studies on this health issue. And not so according to the neighbors. Incidentally, why would it have to be anger directed at a mate—couldn't it just as well be anger directed toward one's job? People who harbor prejudice or deep resentment towards a family member may be in this category as well. Wouldn't it all still have the same detrimental effect? COOL IT! Easier said than done. We've all heard the expression, *Laughter is the best medicine*, well it may also be said that depression (clinical and otherwise) may be the worst kind of medicine. There are additional studies that have addressed cynicism, anti-social behavior, distrust for people and even frustration with one's position in life, all of which may negatively impact someone's health. *(see Whitehall Study)*

> **Triggered by anxiety and negative impulses, blood pressure rises as adrenalin and toxins are released into the system. Coronary arteries narrow restricting blood flow and increasing a risk of *arterial spasm*. There is also a real possibility of generating fatal heart rhythm disturbances.**

A Dr. Raymond Niaura, Ph.D, described in *Psychosomatic Medicine*, January 2000, how hostility is linked to various health maladies, and specifically how it may affect individual *metabolic factors that are known to predict or imply cardiovascular disease*. "A joyful spirit is like good medicine but a bad spirit dryeth the bones."

## ASPIRIN AND ANGER

Here again is a study supporting yet another advantage in taking aspirin. M.D.s James E. Muller, Chief of Cardiovascular, at *Deaconess Hospital/Harvard Medical*, and Murray A. Mittleman, and their associates from 55 medical centers throughout the U.S., found aspirin did *indeed lessen the chances of having a heart attack after a bout of anger*. Statistically, they found an almost 50% risk reduction among those who took aspirin as compared to those who had not.

There was a 2.3 *higher* risk following an
episode of anger for the non-aspirin users as
compared to a 1.3 times *lesser* risk for those in
the study who used aspirin.

# Chapter 32

# Angioplasty *is* *not* **Without Risk**

The *American Heart Association* and the *American College of Cardiology* in 1988, recognizing a degree of patient risk with this procedure, intervened to set guidelines to minimize that risk. The two advisory bodies determined that there was a greater risk to patients among cardiologists and hospitals who had not performed an adequate number of the procedures previously. The organizations suggested what would be the necessary required threshold for individual physician certification with regard to their experience and competence with this procedure.

Originally, they determined a physician must perform no less than 50 angioplasty procedures per year for accreditation. Four years later the number of required performed procedures was raised to 75 per year.

The HIN's article was appropriately entitled, *Practice Makes Perfect In Angioplasty* and reported on two newer studies which had identified specific information that further supported the notion, there was indeed a greater risk to the patient when less experienced physicians performed this invasive procedure.

> The results of these studies more than suggest that the patient and doctor be proactive in qualifying *both the hospital and the physician* who would be performing the procedures.

Here most definitely is a procedure that is almost an art form. The number of patient's angioplasty procedures analyzed would amount to more than 110,000 between the two studies. One of the studies was headed by a Dr. Stephen Ellis from the *Cleveland Clinic Foundation* and included the cooperation of 5 separate medical centers. The findings of the one-year study proved very important, and served to establish for the patient that this procedure is not a "no-brainer" and not one without risk.

> There was a one-in-ten-time complication among those cardiologists who performed less than 70 angiograms during a year, which amounted to a serious 9.3% rate of yearly complication.

Dr. Ellis however, found a much lower (2.9%) complication rate among those physicians who performed 270 or more procedures yearly. The other study, whose lead author was Dr. James Jollis, was the *Duke Study*, in which it was determined that angioplasty procedures performed by doctors 25 or less times per year had a much more significant failure rate than those done by doctors who performed 50 or more in a given year. The doctor in the report cited both a higher death rate from the procedure and the need for emergency open-heart intervention as a result of a botched angioplasty. Whenever this "harmless" procedure is performed, a team of physicians are standing by ready to begin emergency interventional surgery immediately should the need arise. Penetrating an artery wall is one such complication particularly among high-risk patients with advanced atherosclerosis or arteriosclerosis.

## SUMMARY

If you are being advised to undergo an angioplasty procedure make sure you know if the doctor and the hospital have met the required criteria for performed procedures and you have done your due diligence according to the information. Be sure the doctor who was hired to do the procedure is the one who shows up at the date and not a less qualified substitute. It does happen.

# Chapter 33

# Cytomegalovirus
## Risk Factor #VI

## INFLAMMATORY

Don't be surprised that you might have never heard of this next risk factor, not too many people have and yet the evidence implicates it as one of the new risk factors. A very convincing study on CMV and heart disease that included both men and women was published in the *Archives of Internal Medicine*.

> The study determined that of 700 subjects, those with CMV antibodies had a 76% greater chance of developing heart disease over the following five years compared to people who had few or no CMV antibodies.

CMV is another of several infections that can remain active though unnoticed by the carrier, who would not normally have been tested. It is a *viral* infection, whereas chlamidya pneumonaie is bacterial. Viral infections are more difficult to treat as has been obvious in finding cures for two other viral illnesses, cancer and the common cold. The findings of this study indicated that individuals with **diabetes and CMV** had an even greater chance of developing heart disease. Those individuals who harbored a high antibody CMV count in the top 20% showed an increased risk while those with diabetes when coupled with CMV, **had nine times the risk of developing heart disease.** This study was led by *Dr. Paul D. Sorile* of the *National Heart, Lung and Blood Institute* in Bethesda, Maryland. As previously mentioned, certain infections have been associated with the *herpes* family of virus. Included among this illustrious group are *epstein barr*, *herpes simplex* and (CMV), *cytomegalovirus.* Another report by Dr. Stephen E. Epstein, confirmed what we have been studying, and showed that all of these infectious agents are definitely suspect and under extensive investigation as to their contribution to heart disease in general.

## WOMEN AND CMV

An article appearing in the journal *Circulation* explains that there is a difference in the way men and women react to CMV. According to the study, women with antibodies respond differently from an immune standpoint and are more vulnerable to atherosclerosis from previous CMV infection than are their male counterparts.

**CMV is a relatively common infection with as much as 85% of the population in this country having become infected in their lifetimes.**

When one has contracted one or more of these opportunistic infections and they run their normal symptomatic course, bacterium may take an insidious free ride within our bodies and linger in the form of low-grade infection. In this dormant state, they can continue to inflame and damage arteries throughout the entire coronary tree, possibly invading the cerebral areas of the brain. These infections have been identified as risks *independent* of the common risk factors that we normally associate with heart disease. This is new territory and as study continues on inflammatory agents, the direct role of even more infections may be identified and linked to heart disease. Infections and their inflammatory responses are now the subject of concentrated study.

> It is not unreasonable to suggest that in looking for the causes of heart attacks and strokes in people with normal cholesterol, *the search must include a focus on a patient's inflammatory agents such as H. pylori, C pneumonaie, cytomegalovirus and herpes simplex.*

## WHAT IS CONSIDERED HIGH?

Dr. David Siscovick, a professor at the *University of Washington,* reported on a study that included 600 participants, 200 of which had already experienced *a previous myocardial event.* Not only did this study concentrate on *C. pneumonaie,* but like the studies just mentioned also evaluated CMV and *herpes simplex,* the type of herpes normally associated with cold sores.

*The information suggested that those who have been infected from cold sores have twice the propensity for experiencing or even dying from heart disease compared to those who have not been infected.*

**This doesn't mean that anyone who has had a cold sore is going to die of heart disease.** Note: *Cytomegalovirus* and *epstein barr* are both of the herpes family, and while there seems to be more agreement on CMV's role at this date, the jury remains out regarding *epstein barr's* involvement in heart disease. For all intents and purposes, it would seem prudent for a patient with known heart disease to be tested for *C. pneumoniae, CMV, and H. pylori* particularly if they have, as we have discussed, an even slightly elevated HS-CRP reading, (the overall marker for inflammation).

A study presented in an earlier chapter indicated a CRP score of 1.53 brings a *two-fold risk* of heart attack or death. Normally, a score of 5 had been considered the point of beginning concern.

What would be the harm in routinely ordering a $10-$15 CRP evaluation? Still, many physicians will continue going on with business as usual clinging to the old idea that monitoring cholesterol is all that is necessary. They may also say that all this inflammation information has not yet been totally accepted for general application. That is always a safe response and a polite way of dismissing their lack of knowledge or interest in further becoming educated on the subject. Nothing in medicine has been totally, universally accepted until it has been around for many, many years and yet these things we are discussing have been researched for 10 or more years.

> **What about the patient who would benefit from the diagnostics, but who really doesn't have the option of waiting for years until his or her doctor becomes convinced? Why not err on the side of caution in protecting the patient? What would be the downside of testing?**

You or your loved one's healthcare should not be considered an experiment when the leading cardiologists in the country have already accepted such methods in their day-to-day practice. This is the reason so many pharmaceutical houses are bringing their case to you by means of expensive advertising on TV, advising you to talk to your doctor about different medications. Many of the inflammatory conditions just mentioned are in fact among those that comprise the inflammatory risk factors.

*Unless the physician is prepared to concentrate on the entire profile, using all the new testing available, many patients' risk profiles will probably fall through the cracks.*

We could probably agree that no doctor could tell if a patient seated across the desk is or is not HIV or hepatitis C positive without testing their blood. Neither can the doctor identify a patient with a dysfunction in LP (a), ApoB, fibrinogen, or inflammatory illness without testing. Add any of the other risk factors including those influenced by diet and the total risk compounds dramatically. To this dynamic add the possibility of having a present or past infection, as we have been discussing, such as Cp, gum disease and H. pylori, or consider a possible elevated homocysteine level, and the odds mount up against the patient *regardless* of the total cholesterol reading. Factor in diabetes, obesity, mid-body girth, smoking and inadequate physical activity and look out, there is trouble ahead. These additional newly discovered complications demand earlier, more stringent and broader physician diagnostics. The sooner this is the accepted protocol, the fewer cardiovascular and stroke related episodic events will be recorded. We have read that:

*80% OF THESE RISK FACTORS ARE NOT DETECTED DURING THE ROUTINE BLOODWORK DONE ON ONE'S ANNUAL PHYSICAL.*

# Chapter 34

# Deep Vein
# *Thrombosis*

Here is a new term for us to decipher. *Deep Vein Thrombosis* (DVT), which according to the statistics is the FOURTH leading cause of death in the US, affecting one in 1,000 people. It is a phenomenon that occurs when a clot that has formed in the deep recess of one's calf migrates to a vital organ such as a lung or the brain. Studies recently released have identified the scope of the problem and focused on long-range airplane flights, during which a passenger might remain immobile for long periods of time. Especially under threat are those passengers with known circulatory issues on lengthy transcontinental trips.

## BLOOD CLOTS DO KILL
## AIRLINE PASSENGERS

As incredible as it seems, British and Australian doctors have publicly announced that hundreds of passengers each year are affected by blood clots after arriving in their country's airports. According to John Belstead, an emergency consultant at the *Middlesex Ashford Hospital,* these travelers have been meeting their demise at a rate of about one per month. In reporting to *Reuters,* Belstead explained that these individuals had died of a *pulmonary embolism* soon after their arrival at London's Heathrow airport. "These people die as they get off the aircraft," Belstead told the BBC.

## AUSTRALIA WEIGHS IN WITH SIMILAR RESULTS

In Sydney Australia, where passengers arrive after being airborne for very long duration, an estimated 400 people a year (according to an Australian surgeon) become victims of blood clots. It would appear there is a much greater risk among the elderly, and certainly among those individuals dealing with claudication in the legs. Hawaii medical statistics also confirm 69 reported DVT cases over a 7-year period. We have addressed in earlier chapters how many of the elevated viscosity or aggregation markers can complicate the clotting process. Presence of any of these, or a combination of them, would certainly seem to put an individual at even greater risk of DVT episode. People who are obese, smoke, have a history of stroke or hematological problems and those who are not ambulatory are at even greater risk while in flight.

*SOLUTION:* The advice offered is for passengers to get to their feet and walk around from time to time during flight. It is also recommended that passengers periodically perform ankle/foot rotation and foot extensions while in their seats.

# THE TROPONINS:
# TWO LIFESAVING BLOOD TESTS
# FOR ANGINA HEART PATIENTS

There is a cutting-edge test that, a study claims, is able to identify the formation of tiny clots in the subject's blood, thereby fore-warning the physician if a patient might be destined for a heart attack or stroke within the near future. The *troponin T* provides rapid evaluation and is usually performed in a hospital along with other biochemical markers like *creatine kinase* (CK) and *creatine kinase-MB* (CKMB) to assess whether or not a person is actually currently experiencing a heart attack. A study exploring the association between patients with unstable angina and higher levels of *troponin T* was performed at the *University Hospital in Uppsala, Sweden*. When the 975 men and women in the study were tested and their progress monitored, the following was established:

> **Those in the top 1/5th of the scale, recording the higher levels of *Troponin-T*, had a 16.1% risk of falling victim to either a heart attack or dying within the _following five-month period_ compared to 4.3% for those in the lower percentage—an almost four-fold higher risk.**

TROPONIN 1, is used to detect actual cardiac injury, to predict mortality and as a marker for measuring perioperative general heart attack damage.

## SUMMARY

Here is yet another example of a simple blood test that could save the lives of numerous individuals if the test were ordered as a *preventive test for outpatients* and not simply called upon as a marker to establish whether or not someone is having a heart attack at the time of hospital admittance. *If you or someone you know is experiencing angina (compromised blood flow accompanied by chest pain),* **you might encourage them to ask their doctor to prescribe this test as a preventive action.**

# Chapter 35

# *Sudden Death Among* Young People

How big a problem is this phenomenon? According to the *CDC* in the first national study of sudden cardiac death, 23,320 young people were lost in just the seven-year period from 1989 to 1996. These startling numbers were retrieved from nation-wide death certificate records of young people between 15 and 34 years of age. Twenty-one percent of these subjects were actually under 24. This according to Dr. Zhi-Jie Zheng, M.D., Ph.D. The study author was alarmed at the number of young girls affected, and believed that early smoking and teenage obesity may have played a part.

---

**According to the CDC, sudden cardiac death claimed the lives of 3,000 young adults who had appeared to be in good health.**

---

# HEART ATTACKS AMONG YOUNG ATHLETES

We have all heard of athletes who have experienced heart attacks while performing in their respective sports. The entire world was shocked when a 24-year-old Olympic pairs ice-skating champion, Sergey Gordeeva, died during one of his regularly scheduled workouts several years ago. In June of 2000, 33-year-old Cardinal pitcher Darryl Kile died in his sleep. It was later determined that Kile had two occluded coronary arteries, one 80% and the other 90%. Young athletes dying in the prime of life from America's number one killer, heart disease. Haven't you wondered about such cases? Remember the three young basketball players who dropped dead during their basketball games? How about Hank Gathers? The news has carried similar reports in recent years of several football players who died on the field of play. Kory Stringer was one such athlete whose death immediately comes to mind. Someone sent me an obituary that appeared in a major New York newspaper. The deceased individual, whose name appeared in the column, was a former champion runner who had experienced a heart attack during one of his daily runs. Whenever we learn of a heart attack crisis that befalls an outstanding athlete, we are taken aback. It just isn't supposed to happen this way. People who exercise, maintain their weight and lower their cholesterol are not supposed to be taken by heart disease! And yet we hear of it happening over and over again. Why? Hopefully there are some explanations in what you are about to read that may help you divert an otherwise health-threatening crisis, particularly among your youngsters involved in athletics.

# ONE FAMILY'S
# TRAGEDY

Chuck Morrell is doing well seven years after his heart transplant. Chuck and his twin brother Gary were both superb college football players at Washington State University. Chuck is the lucky twin who remains a survivor of *Hypertrophic Cardiomyopathy* (HCM). This is a critically serious genetic disease whose impact too often affects the families of young people—more specifically, to families of young athletes. **The Morrell family lost five immediate members to this tragic disease.** To see just how indiscriminate this killer can be, just look at the various ways it impacted this one family. Chuck's half-sister, Michelle, died in her sleep at 3 years of age, Chuck's mother Virginia at 54, his twin brother's son Kyle died at 12 to be followed six months later by his 14 year old brother Mitchell. Mitchell's sister, Chuck's niece, Desiree went into full cardiac arrest walking home from school when she (like her brother before her) was just 14 years of age. Thankfully, two fellow students intervened performing CPR until paramedics arrived and revived her. (This is, incidentally, another example of why CPR training should be encouraged at all levels.) Desiree went on to raise a son, Tyler, who at age 11 was also diagnosed with HCM and had an I.C.D. (*defibrillator*) implanted. Tyler is currently doing well with the protection of the device. Finally, Chuck's 54-year-old twin brother Gary Morrell became the fifth member of the Morrell family to fall victim to HCM. Gary died at age 54. Chuck Morrell himself was given a heart transplant at UCLA in 1995. As we prepare to go to press in 2003 Chuck informs me that his oldest daughter Holly has now also been diagnosed with HCM and a *defibrillator* has since been implanted. Holly did not exhibit a thickening of the heart wall as did the other family members but was found to carry a newly recognized HCM defective gene. Their story belongs here because many of these deaths might have been averted if preventive measures and diagnostics had been applied. Most victims of HCM expire similarly as did the members of the Morrell family. Many youngsters taken by this illness died while performing in competitive events without any prior warning. Several other victims died shortly after their games were over and in some cases, during actual pre-game warm-ups and drills. Basketball star Hank Gathers was just 23 when he died during a basketball tournament. A 20-year-old Kansas State football player died while driving his car. Louis Savino became a victim of HCM during a routine game of soccer when he was only 15. A 16-year-old young man named Scotty Lang of Orange, CA lost his life during football practice. **The *Minneapolis Heart Institute Foundation* several years ago recorded the statistic that 43 high school and college level athletes had become victims of HCM.** Nineteen were basketball players, twenty were football players, four track competitors, one played soccer, one tennis, and one was a swimmer. You can see from this cross-section that if your youngster is involved in any sport there may be a small but real risk. To be more specific, any child, whether or not they are involved in competitive sports, may still have this time bomb ticking within their chest. How many young people have died over the past 100 years whose families did not have the benefit of an autopsy performed to determine the direct cause? No one was keeping score. **How would you as a parent know if your child is currently at risk for HCM?** We will never know how many lives this form of heart disease stole in past years but there is something that can be done today to identify a child at risk. The *American Heart Association,* acknowledging the danger to youngsters as proved by the many deaths to athletes, presented a set of guidelines and recommendations for pre-screening student athletes at the high school and college levels. **Today, six years later, student athletes are still dying in the course of on-field or on-court competition. The guidelines (in many cases) have been ignored because of the added expense of implementing (cardiac ultrasound) testing.** *Hypertrophic Cardiomyopathy* (HCM) delivers its destruction by causing a thickening of the heart muscle itself affecting the wall that separates the ventricles, obstructing blood flow and facilitating the development of an *erratic* heart beat which too often culminates in *sudden death.*

> **HCM is the leading cause of death in this country among people, and particularly young athletes, affecting one in 500 people.**

When the overall causes of loss of life is segmented among young, 36% is awarded to HCM. Chuck Morrell's story doesn't end here; he has been involved with the formation of an organization called *A Heart for Sports,* which is hell-bent on educating parents and family members about this devastating disease, and making sure their youngster is evaluated before it becomes too late. The organization *A Heart For Sports* was founded through the dedication and commitment of *Seaneen Greaves* and her co-founder husband *Jeff,* and they are making a difference. Their personal story and additional information regarding their organization may be found at their website (*www.aheartforsports.org).* Seaneen, Jeff and Chuck would be the first to advise parents to be proactive in asking their child's coaches if their youngster had been properly evaluated by *echocardiogram* (ultrasound) for this ailment. Better yet, if your child's school hasn't been able to provide the necessary $800-$1,500 cost of an evaluation, students and parents might choose to become involved in various fundraising activities to acquire the money for an actual echocardiogram machine to be purchased for their athletic departments. Smaller versions of these machines can be affordable, and are available for around $3,000, although the upgraded versions range upwards to $22,000 and even $250,000. These echocardiogram tests can mean the difference between life and death for a youngster. *A Heart For Sports* recently met with the organization of echo cardiographers (sonographers) who pledged a desire to perform these ultrasound evaluations for little or no compensation. This disease needs to be identified at the earliest school level.

## SUMMARY

Think of the possibilities if the NFL and the NBA got involved, making donations to school athletic programs in their franchise areas and promoting public awareness? After all, their future athletes come to them from the high school and college ranks. They have more than a passing interest in sports. Certain parents might themselves choose to pay to have the exam administered by the family doctor, if their insurance doesn't cover the test. Hank Gather's death might never have happened, nor so many of the other deaths we have heard about, if an ultrasound had been performed many years earlier by an alert athletic program and a defibrillator had been implanted.

# Chapter 36

# FRAMINGHAM,
## *the* *Gold Standard* Study

In 1948, the landmark $43 million, ten-year *Framingham Heart Study* confirmed, defined and established cholesterol's role in heart disease. A forty-three million dollar budget fifty years ago was a lot of money! Never before or since has there been a study that would have as far-reaching and revolutionary an effect. Michael DeBakey, world-renowned heart surgeon, was later inspired to say, *"It has set the model in epidemiology. It is truly one of the great studies of this century."* The study among its many other findings debunked the misguided belief that blood pressure elevations were an *automatic* result of aging as had been the accepted theory. However the study would further prove that high blood pressure was indeed still a risk factor for heart disease. The study also provided data in 1974 that proved diabetes certainly complicated the cardiovascular risk profile. Basically, this major study separated fact from fiction. It conflicted and countered much of the previously accepted science and thereby wrote its own revolutionary chapter. It is still writing it more than fifty years later. One might have expected the medical community at large to have accepted and embraced the study's findings openly, immediately applying the information. But many physicians 15 or more years after the information was released in 1977 were still remaining obstinate about ordering HDL, LDL and triglyceride evaluations. Many agreed to test, but only the one <u>total overall cholesterol test.</u> It was Framingham that informed the profession in 1983 that a condition called *mitral valve prolapse* was a risk to be evaluated in patients. Doctors suddenly began paying more attention to this dysfunction. In the same year, **fibrinogen was found by the study to cause an increased risk in heart disease.** Framingham also determined in 1988 that something called HDL cholesterol was to be considered beneficial. It was announced earlier in 1987 that high levels of cholesterol had a direct association with premature death among young men, and in 1989 cigarette smoking was finally linked with stroke. Four years later Framingham reported on how even mildly elevated systolic blood pressure increased the risk of heart disease, and the next year brought the news that genes like LP (a) and ApoE (which we will begin to hear more of) were implicated as risk factors. There are many, many more groundbreaking findings that have come out of this famous study. There is today also a substantial body of evidence that takes up where Framingham left off. A newer generation of advanced application has sprung from much of the earlier data that contributed to the original findings. Researchers have been probing even deeper into the cholesterol framework, identifying inherited factors that have only recently begun to receive well-deserved attention. They have been hard at work exploring other sources which contribute to heart disease that were not recognized or at least not accepted 10, 5 or even 3 years ago. These new findings, supported by the evidence which you are reading, offer a deeper look into the complicated cardiovascular heart disease maze. Areas of research for our benefit and certainly our children's are continually being advanced including chromosome and genes that bring dysfunction in hypertension or high cholesterol. Still, based on the record of how long it has taken for doctors in general to finally accept the recommendations of the original Framingham study, one has to wonder how many doctors 10-20 years from now will still be resisting the newest information and trial results, or if they will embrace them to the benefit of their patients. Some will, some won't. Your job is to find one who takes the new information seriously and will apply it to diagnosing and treating your family.

# Chapter 37

# Snoring
## and *Sleep Apnea*
### more than just an annoyance

S leep apnea can be a very serious, life-threatening ailment and should be acknowledged as such among heart disease patients. There are mixed reports concerning the number of people who expire in their sleep because of sleep apnea. Certain statistics suggest the number is more than 1,500 a year, while others speculate 2,500 and are quick to add that the number may be many more. The reason it is difficult to ascertain the actual mortality figures is that when someone dies during their sleep from any form of heart disease, it is assumed they died of a heart attack, and the case is filed and closed. Their heart has stopped and therefore the final cause is attributed to sudden death or cardiac arrest which is in fact accurate. **In truth, they could have died as a direct cause of complications set in motion by one of two forms of sleep apnea, central or obstructive.** There are degrees of this dysfunction in which the person literally stops breathing as many as 200 or more times a night, depriving the individual of necessary sleep. These individuals awake tired, often falling asleep during their work hours or simply struggle to keep awake. In order to enter the most advantageous level of sleep, called *Delta* (the third level), one needs to have been sleeping uninterruptedly for several hours. A person with apnea is awakened repeatedly, as they gasp for a breath of air to survive. The true way of diagnosing this illness is to submit to an overnight sleepover in a sleep deprivation clinic. This can be expensive and uncomfortable.

## WHEN SMALL CHILDREN SNORE

According to the new guidelines and advice from the American Academy of Pediatrics, sleep apnea may be a concern for parents whose young children snore. Doctor Carole Marcus, director of *Johns Hopkins University Pediatric Sleep Center,* has given the following advice.

*" Parents should be aware that snoring is not necessarily a normal phenomenon for their children and they should discuss it with their doctors. "*

This *obstructive sleep apnea* condition is one that has been under-diagnosed and has only recently been identified as a factor that poses risk. The study statistics suggest that half a million young people between ages 2-8 are the most affected. If the truth were known through proper diagnosis, many youngsters displaying learning problems as attention deficit are actually having difficulty in concentration from a lack of sleep. They are simply exhausted and often show signs of irritability that causes teachers to label them "difficult children to handle." The researchers are quick to point out that a physician would first want to consider enlarged tonsils or adenoids as the cause of the breathing difficulty before arriving at a sleep apnea diagnosis. These first-time assembled guidelines can be found in the 4/2002 issue of the *American Academy of Pediactrics*. The advice from *Johns Hopkins* alerts parents that if their child shows heavy open-mouthed breathing, snores or has demonstrations of apnea during sleep, it would be prudent to address these concerns with the child's doctor. The adult snorer and the youngster have much in common. Both have difficulty in maintaining focus. The child dozes off in class, and the adult finds it difficult to maintain concentration and be effective in his or her work. There is also a too real danger of falling asleep behind the wheel.

A study on adults entitled *Sleep Apnea in 81 Ambulatory Male Patients With Stable Heart Failure* by Javaheri, Liming and colleagues appeared in *Circulation* 1998. This study of sleep apnea and the result of repetitive asphyxia found that it has an **adverse affect on the actual function of the heart.** The patients recruited for the study had been diagnosed with heart failure and had been recorded with a low left ventricle ejection output of 45%. Briefly, the study found that patients with this disorder have a high amount of atrial fibrillation and ventricular arrhythmias, both as we have studied, are very serious disorders. Other studies have shown this condition among heart failure patients to be more serious than had been previously acknowledged.

**The left ventricle enlarges weakening over time and is often the cause of "sudden death." Sleep apnea can be a very serious ailment.**

A wife can give her husband a pretty good idea of how long the episodes between breaths last in duration and how often they occur. God knows she isn't able to sleep anyway. Women of course also snore, as sleep apnea is not a gender-based ailment. **A study reported in the *American Journal of Epidemiology* in mid 2002 involving 70,000 nurses claimed that women snorers release a hormone that creates a pathway to *insulin resistance*, which can predispose them to type 2 diabetes.** How can you be sure you are or are not a serious snorer? I suggested an inexpensive first method of evaluation to a friend who needed to hear for himself how severe his snoring had become. He bought a $25 small *voice activated* tape recorder. It would only activate during the periods of snoring, and when he awoke he had the wonderful experience of hearing himself for about a solid hour, which might have been a whole night's actual snoring. He learned two things from the experience.

Firstly, that his wife must really love him to sleep in the same room as a snorer who sounds like a freight train. Secondly, in playing the tape for his doctor, he learned he definitely had a potentially dangerous medical condition. Overweight is one of the most obvious reason for apnea. When one gains weight that shows itself on the exterior of the neck and throat area, the weight is also gained internally within the area that affects the space between the tongue the soft palate and pharynx. With time the added weight and the "veils" (the soft tissue on either side of the back of the throat), lose some elasticity and encroach upon the air pathway. There are numerous snoring aids on the market. There are also surgeries. One removes most of the uvula, that little finger that is visible at the back of the throat when you look in the mirror. Some get relief from this procedure and some don't. Another surgery corrects those "veils" just mentioned. There is a newer use of the technology of radio frequency, which was studied and tested at *Stanford University*. This radio frequency procedure actually reduces the thickness in the center of the tongue itself at the rear of the throat. Apparently the procedure avoids the sides of the tongue where the nerve endings reside. According to the clinical studies, the meaty part of the organ may be reduced up to 21%, such reduction permits more airway. There is also the issue of allergies, which compromise the ability to breath through one's nose during sleep, resulting in open-mouth breathing, which sets apnea in motion. If you awaken in the morning with a dry mouth you can pretty well deduce that you have been breathing through your mouth. In all fairness, diuretics and certain allergy medications can produce this negative effect as well. The *Breathe Right* nasal strips you see on NFL football players and other athletes actually bring a degree of relief for many snorers, and might be considered the first line of defense before trying anything else. You don't have to be an NFL athlete to benefit from these little strips and amazingly they really do provide benefit. In literally thousands of cases this breathing aid is all that is needed.

# Chapter 38

# Matters of the HEART

### Cardiac arrest, Ventrical dysfunction, Atrial fibrillation

Perhaps you have heard a story similar to this one. A wife is busy in the kitchen while her husband is watching television in the living room. The woman speaks to her husband from the kitchen, but he doesn't respond. She walks into the adjoining room where he appears to be napping, but decides against disturbing his slumber. When he hasn't awakened after a normal period of time, she nudges him, only to find that his slumber has become permanent. He had become another victim of cardiac arrest. Had there been symptoms that could have been detected earlier? Cardiac arrest is most often the result of suspected or *unsuspected* underlying heart disease. In 90% of cases, two or more major coronary arteries have been compromised by atheroclerosis. Sudden death, as the term suggests, can strike without warning. The AHA instructs an immediate call to 911 and the beginning of CPR, as the patient's chance of survival without intervention will decrease 7-10% with each passing minute and time is of the essence. If emergency services arrive within 5-7 minutes to begin defibrillation, there is an approximately 49% success rate in reviving the victim. Sudden death is sometimes referred to as *sudden cardiac arrest* or *unexpected cardiac arrest*. Here are the study statistics presented at the *American Heart Association's* 41st annual conference on Cardiovascular Disease Epidemiology and Prevention.

> **Cardiac arrest remains the cause of 259,000 deaths a year in this country alone. One half of those who die of heart disease succumb within one hour of the noticeable symptoms.**

Twenty-five to thirty-three percent of those who suffer sudden cardiac death die instantly, and unless the event has occurred in the presence of others, the victim is usually found after the fact quite by accident. The lucky ones are those within the remaining percentage of patients, who experience symptoms and are able to get to a hospital to take advantage of emergency care. The statistics report that about one half of CHD deaths each year are attributed to sudden death cases, accounting for more than 680 people per day. The AMA and the AHA advise learning the symptoms, and not hesitating to act if you or someone you know are displaying symptoms. If you are within range of paramedic services, call. If not have someone take you to the hospital due haste. It would not be wise to go to sleep waiting to see if the symptoms are still there in the morning. It is possible that something as simple as indigestion may ultimately turn out to be the cause, but to their own detriment *a lot of people have delayed seeking medical attention, misdiagnosing their own symptoms.* **Tomorrow isn't** promised to anyone, and the prudent approach is better, wouldn't you agree? There is no doubt the graveyards are hosting a few too many guests who thought they simply might have eaten a little too much pasta and could have "slept it off." Some of them are still sleeping! Why risk the gamble? As the old advice suggests, "better to be safe than sorry!" While it is a fact that many people expire without previous indications or symptoms, the warning signs that indicate the potential consequence could very often have been detected earlier. **Ninety percent of cases of Sudden Cardiac Death** are the result of heart disease which is known to have been detectable. EBCT or treadmill anyone?

# THE CAUSES

Causes include a previous heart attack which resulted in acquired damaged scar tissue or even death to certain portions of the heart muscle itself. A history of hypertension and even rheumatic fever earlier in someone's life can definitely be root causes of this killer. Damaged areas of the heart serve as poor conductors of the electrical currents received from the atrium control center, and short circuit or even misdirect electrical current. In cardiac arrest (myocardial infarction) the heart literally stops beating. According to the *American Medical Association*, it is usually finally caused by disruption of the rhythm to one or both of the lower ventricles, a malfunction often involving ventricle fibrillation (not to be confused with atrial fibrillation which occurs in the upper atrium). In cases of *atrial fibrillation*, where the problem exists in the artrium rather than the ventricle, there is an *increase of stroke* as much as five-fold.

*Ventricle fibrillation* happens if the muscles that control the ventricles of the two lower chambers of the heart *spasm* or "twitch" out of coordination, causing the heart to cease pumping blood to the brain and the rest of the body. Cardiac arrest is too often the final result. The chapter exalting the preventive benefits of fish oil is very relevant to this form of rhythmic disease.

## THE "WIDOW MAKER"

*Statistics support the fact that as many as 90% of heart attacks involve the left ventricle.* It is the heart's main pumping chamber and has the dubious distinction of being called the "Widow Maker." It is the muscular chamber of the heart that accepts blood from the left atrium (upper chamber) and ejects or releases the blood into the aorta. It is here in this process that the *ejection fraction* is recorded during one's nuclear test. The ejection fraction is a measurement of how effectively the heart is able to function as it sends the blood back through the system. Physicians will often order an echocardiogram to measure the ventricle wall for thickness and size. Negative results when found may have been caused by uncontrolled elevated blood pressure. Your cardiologist may also be concerned with leakage as a result of calcification or stenosis to a valve or the valve leaflets. Regurgitation of a diseased aortic or mitral valve literally causes the reversal of blood flow back from the leaking valve. This is a serious process that we discussed in an earlier chapter, and one which causes the left ventricle to enlarge from the extra load put upon it as the heart "over pumps" to compensate for the diminished blood flow. The danger here is that even when the valve is replaced or repaired with a mechanical or animal valve, the damage to the ventricle will permanently have deprived it of some of its ability to function.

# HEART VALVE DISEASE

▶ **Aortic Valve Sclerosis** is a condition occurring when calcium deposits become encrusted on the valve leaflets causing them to become thick and inflexible. This condition is mostly found in patients in their mid-sixties. It is accompanied by a *systolic* heart murmur diagnosed by a physician listening with a stethoscope to the sound of escaping air at the second *intercostal* space located below the breast or sternum bone. This is not a very uncommon disease, however, patients identified with this disease have about a 50% increased risk of cardiovascular problems compared to those without the diagnosis. Aortic sclerosis is a different disease than aortic stenosis. Aortic stenosis often progresses to the second and advanced disease when the patient develops angina and heart failure. In cases where calcification of the valve presents in patients under 40 the most common cause would have been congenital and present at birth. Minor findings of calcification do not usually require treatment.

▶ **Aortic Valve Stenosis** In this disease it is not the leaflets that are the concern it is the actual valve that becomes calcified and narrowed. These patients typically are out of breath and easily tired as the heart must work extra hard in forcing blood through the diseased valve.

▶ **Valve Regurgitation** is a serious disease in which the valve becomes so diseased by calcification and scarring that it is unable to open and close sufficiently permitting the blood to flow backwards through the valve. We have all seen what happens when a faucet valve in the kitchen sink becomes worn. The water continues to flow even though the faucet itself has been tightly closed. There are four heart valves: **Aortic, Mitral, Bicuspid and Tricuspid.**

## YOUR AMAZING HEART

• It is a muscle about the size of your fist.

• It pumps 100,000 times a day.

• 2,000 gallons in a 24 hour day.

• In a 70 year lifespan it pumps 2.5 billion times.

• All the blood vessels involved in your circulatory system laid end to end would encircle the earth more than two times.

In case you think there is nothing about you special, know that your little heart will pump enough blood in your lifetime to fill 3½ oil tankers!

## THE HEART'S CONSTRUCTION

The heart has four chambers with the command center positioned in the right atrium. The purpose of the command center is to control the critical electrical impulses that dictate the timing of contractions to all chambers of the heart. Not unlike the way the distributor of an automobile sends out electrical impulses to the spark plugs. A "mis-fire" may offset the natural rhythm of the heart's chambers, producing catastrophic effect. The general reasons for disease in these areas of rhythm are grounded in actual heart disease, but there is another potential cause, and that lies with patients who have earlier in their lives experienced *Rheumatic fever*. Most frequently however, the information confirms that the problem is the result of advancing heart disease. How well a physician is able to read and interpret the many subtle indications recorded on EKG tests is one example of how levels of competence between practitioners can differ. An EKG reading, properly, accurately interpreted by a talented observer can reveal a warning easily overlooked by someone less observant or less capable. Malcom Thaler's book on EKG is a real education.

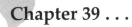

# Chapter 39

# *Inhibitors*

Several new drugs are being employed to regress left ventricle hypertrophy (enlargement). One is *Altace* (Ramipril), another *Enalapril* in the ACE *(angiotensin-converting enzyme)* inhibitor class. Both have shown outstanding results. *Altace* has proven to be one of those drugs that provides added benefit for heart failure patients beyond simply modifying high blood pressure values. This drug has proven concurrently to provide remarkable advantage against other ailments, including diabetic neuropathy. The findings of multiple uses for certain drugs is a phenomenon that occurs often. As example, *monoxidil* was originally developed as a blood pressure medication, and yet it was coincidentally found to be effective in growing hair. Another blood pressure medication, *Hytrin*, was added to the arsenal of weapons in treating prostate disease. The medical profession took a real serious look at *Altace* when a January 2000 edition of the *New England Journal of Medicine* reported amazing statistics from the *Hope Trial* (Heart

Outcomes Prevention Evaluation), regarding this ACE inhibitor in it's class of drugs known as angiotensin enzyme converting drugs. As *Altace* was proving itself an effective therapy for what it was originally intended, (hypertension), it also dramatically **reduced patient death from *all* causes by 16%**! It is necessary to add that other ACE inhibitor drugs have shown similar benefit by inhibiting angiotensin production, but this article's concentration was singularly on *Altace*. Here are the results of the study, which involved 9,297 subjects over age 55. The participants took either this drug or a placebo for a period of five years, and the following is what all the excitement has been about.

## THE HOPE TRIAL

When the patients in the two groups were compared in this international trial, the *Altace*, group had exhibited a **25% less chance of a person dying** from *any* cardiovascular event compared to the placebo group. Further, the members of the *Altace* group were **20%** *less* **likely** to have experienced a heart attack. The study also concluded that patients in this group were **31%** *less likely to suffer a stroke* than the placebo group plus a 61% reduced risk of fatal stroke. The reported benefits do not end here, as there was also a **37%** *reduction in sudden death* cases from *rhythm disturbance*. Now, try this one...there was a **16%** *reduction* in the trial for needing angioplasty or bypass surgeries among the *Altace* group. This angiotensin class of drugs operates by blocking the production of a hormone known as *angiotensin II*. There is speculation that other ACE inhibitor drugs might have also proven similar benefits had they been put through the same trial standard as the HOPE study, however that would remain to be seen. Incidentally, the HOPE was not a trial designed to just study blood pressure medications. Those patients diagnosed with peripheral vascular disease (PAD) and those presenting with coronary artery disease (CAD), heart failure, diabetes, and/or related diabetic neuropathy, might want to confer with their doctor as to whether this drug class and this particular drug would provide additional benefit for their particular condition and overall chances of survival. Data from the HOPE study indicated a significant 25 to 30 percent reduction in the risk of death from cardiovascular disease *among diabetics*. Diabetes and heart disease conflicting the same patient is a combination difficult to treat, however these study findings should be welcome news. Coming out of the 2001 annual *Sessions of The American Heart Association* was information that the ACE Inhibitors have shown a very strong ability to control *inflammation* factors, and this may provide yet another explanation as to how this class of drug might be contributing to the reduction of heart attacks. In 2003 the growing interest in inflammatory factors make this finding even more important. Blood pressure control may actually prove to be the least of the benefits. One of the potential drawbacks of the ACE inhibitors is that some patients develop an annoying chest cough. Another is a negative correlation which might occur among heart failure patients taking an ACE inhibitor drug and aspirin. Independent studies have suggested that pulmonary activity among these particular patients may suffer as a result. Clinical tests have also indicated that aspirin may (among certain HF patients) disturb pulmonary activity related to gas exchange, general exercise, peak exercise and oxygen uptake levels. The amount of ASA monitored daily through the Milan, Italy study was 325 mgs. How smaller amounts of daily

ASA would affect these exercise and pulmonary outcomes was not determined in the particular study. Your doctor will evaluate and determine on a case-by-case basis whether or not the benefits outweigh the risks with each individual patient. *Altace* (as discussed above) **was shown to reduce the risk of dying from "sudden death" by a considerable 37 percent,** as reported in the *Study of Left Ventricle Dysfunction,* (SOLVD). Treating patients with *enalapril,* a different ACE inhibitor, did reduce death from cardiovascular disease by a significant 18% as well as providing a 22% reduction in death cases among heart failure patients. **By way of comparison, *Altace* posted a 37% reduction in this protocol, according to the study.**

Angiotensin-Converting Enzyme Inhibitor therapy update: A recent study documented improvement of a serious heart ailment: Left Ventricular Hypertrophy (LVH). The study attributed regression of the disease to Altace (Ramipril).

# Chapter 40

# DIURETICS *verse*

## *other* Blood Pressure Medications

▶ A study released in the *New England Journal of Medicine* in late 2002 brought new focus to *diuretic* blood pressure medications. The study compared this class of hypertensive medication to commonly used but more expensive medications. No doubt insurance companies will like this study, as many of these diuretic drugs are generic and inexpensive. Diuretics serve to lower blood pressure by removing sodium and excess water from the blood and tissues. Lasix is often prescribed for congestive heart failure to remove excess buildup of water around the heart and ankles resulting from left ventricle inefficiency. Like all medications, there are advantages and disadvantages to be weighed in providing the best therapy for the patient. Diuretics can affect electrolytes and the sodium potassium balance, which is critical to heart function. Patients with arrhythmic disorders need to be monitored carefully as low electrolyte levels can set off erratic heartbeat. Patients on diuretic therapy must be aware not to spend prolonged time in the sun because of the depleted fluid from the skin. These drugs are used very effectively in *combination* with other hypertensive drugs for certain patients. Doctors have been cautioned about a possible interaction among post-angioplasty patients when a combination of an ACE inhibitor is commonly prescribed with aspirin or the non-steroidal type inflammatory aids of the *Advil* or *Ibuprofen* type. In a study presented at the *American College of Cardiology* in 3/ 1999 there was evidence of a 3-fold increased mortality rate among the patients in the study who were administered the combination compared to patients taking aspirin alone.

## COMMON CLASSES OF HYPERTENSIVE DRUGS

Each of these classes of medication was developed for different heart and blood pressure problems.

▶ ACE INHIBITORS, block *angiotensin I and II* by interfering with the body's production of the *angiotensin-converting enzyme* which contributes to high blood pressure and reduces heart attack. This class of drug is also used effectively for congestive heart failure. The preceding entry on *Altace and the HOPE study* explained many additional advantages offered by this drug. These are four members of this class: *Cozarr, Zestrel, Lotensin, Prinivil.*

▶ CALCIUM CHANNEL BLOCKERS are prescribed for angina, hypertension and arrhythmias. They dilate blood vessels lowering the heart's demand for oxygen. CCB drugs also slow down the heart's workload by dilating blood vessels and controlling calcium distribution to cell membranes. A few are, *Calan, Carizem, Norvasc, Procardia.*

▶ BETA-BLOCKERS are of the *beta-adrenergic* blocking class of drug. They reduce the amount of oxygen needed by the heart by slowing the rate of heartbeat. They serve as antiarrhythmic and antihypertensive drugs, and are often prescribed for patients suffering from palpitations or symptoms induced by anxiety. *Altenolol, Inderal, Lopressor* are all beta-blockers and are prescribed for CAD, angina and heart failure. They slow heart rate reducing the heart workload, lower blood pressure, stabilize heart rhythms and reduce the risk of a second heart attack.

▶ ALPHA ADRENERGIC BLOCKERS (alpha blockers) dilate blood vessels. Three such drugs are *Hytrin, Flomax and Cardura.*

▶ DIURETICS are effective for reducing edema in the legs and lungs by deporting sodium through the urine. There are many including *Thiazides, Diuril, Hygroton, Furosemide, Hyrodiuril, and Hydrodyizide.*

## SUMMARY

While much is currently being written about diuretics, there are individual reasons why each of the three classes of drugs just discussed were developed. As effective as diuretics can be in controlling blood pressure, denying the positive benefits of a particular drug for a less expensive generic diuretic, may not be in the best interest of the patient. There are certain drugs and one called *Zestoretic*, which incorporates the advantages of an ACE inhibitor and a diuretic in one application. A diuretic called *Triamterene* is a drug in the *potassium sparing class* that does not require potassium supplementation. Most patients on diuretics are advised to include a banana or orange juice in their daily diet to provide the necessary potassium. Both are fairly high caloric additions to one's diet. Diet conscious individuals may choose to supplement with Potassium Gluconate.

# Chapter 41

# Congestive Heart Failure
## *(an epidemic)*

It would appear that the description of heart failure as "epidemic in proportion" is accurate, as more and more of the general population reach 65 years of age. There is even more need today for concentration on maintaining the cardiovascular health of this senior population with the increasing number of patients. **Statistically, five million Americans are currently coping with this condition with more than 650,000 new cases added to the rolls each year.** Projections by some sources show an increase of 46% or 6.9 million cases by 2004. The condition known more formerly as *congestive heart failure* can affect people of all ages, although those over 65 are among the most common victims. The cost for physician care, standard treatment and hospital admissions in the U.S. alone might reach 30 billion with the disease accounting for 5%-10% of all hospital admissions. Many patients are hoping and praying for a donor heart to arrive in time. There is a critical shortage, and for those that do become available there is an age limitation. Technology is working to provide temporary mechanical hearts for patients who otherwise would not survive as they wait for a heart to become available. These devices can only provide a short-term fix, if one is even able to obtain one.

## HEART FAILURE: ITS CAUSE

Fundamentally, when someone is diagnosed with heart failure the heart is not able to function nearly to the capacity that it once did. This is the final result of abuse to one's body, perhaps by neglect of the very issues that contributed to the advanced degree of atherosclerosis. The heart may also have become damaged by a prolonged untreated condition of high blood pressure, in other cases heart valves may have sustained damage from a genetic birth condition. The problem often is the result of an inflammatory disease such as endocarditis or myocarditis or very frequently rheumatic fever. Each of these three infections have been identified as contributors to heart failure. A previous experience with heart attack itself scars the tissue and heart muscle affecting the heart's very ability to function at full capacity. At this point in the progression, the heart is losing its ability to adequately fill and empty the ventricles, the opinions of the attending physicians would support a diagnosis of congestive heart failure.

## HOW CHF AFFECTS ONE'S LIFE

We know the heart is the life pump that supplies life-sustaining oxygen and as the heart begins to fail, everyday tasks and enjoyments involving even the slightest exertion, become more taxing and exhausting. The heart does not meet the needs one's body is calling upon it to fulfill. In short, the right ventricle (which supplies the blood to the lungs) and the left ventricle (that feeds the remainder of the body) are failing in their appointed functions.

**THE DEGREE OF DEPRESSION OF LEFT VEN-TRICULAR EJECTION FRACTION (LVEF) IS THE SINGLE MOST POWERFUL PREDICTOR OF SUD-DEN CARDIAC DEATH, AND IT IS EVEN MORE POWERFUL WITH THE ONSET OF CONGESTIVE HEART FAILURE.**

It is a progressive disease that eventually affects one's every normal activity; climbing a short flight of stairs or even walking can become a monumental task. The body becomes starved for oxygen as demands are put upon the weakened organ. The *lung function* becomes compromised as fluid builds, reducing the lung's ability to pump fresh oxygen, which further weakens the heart muscle. A spiraling decline is in process. *When the kidneys* lose more of their ability to perform their normal tasks a combination of cardiac/renal disease begins. *Edema* (water retention) in the legs and lungs become an ever-present consequence.

**This information is meant to prevent you or a loved one from ever coming to this fork in the cardiovascular road.**

The same issues that are concerns for the person desiring to maintain cardiovascular health become even more critical to anyone who faces a prognosis of *heart failure.* Anything that now causes the constriction of the arteries and overloads the damaged heart with workload, including displays of anger, physical exertion, obesity or high blood pressure, provide a definite threat of myocardial infarction and "sudden death."

> **Everything you have come to know about preventing and controlling heart disease becomes even more critical once someone has a diagnosis of heart failure.**

Statistically, winter takes its toll on HF patients with a 20% increase in cardiac death in the early winter months of each year compared to the number of deaths in the summer. There is a difference of 35% mortality between the high and low temperature months. The advice the professionals give is to interact with one's doctors during these winter months in monitoring health and minimizing activity. While there is no cure for this ailment there are several medications plus much supportive information I found in the literature identifying certain heart-friendly supplements. These claims have been substantiated in hundreds of clinical studies. The information presented here will hopefully prove informative for purposes of interaction with your physician. Congestive heart failure is a very serious ailment, and rather than embarking on self-treatment programs, the patient must rely on the doctor's knowledge and approval. There may be significant hope for the heart failure patient in the following information from the alternative medical community. Your doctor may have an interest in this information.

# Chapter 42

# SUPPLEMENTS that
# *improve* HEART FUNCTION

## COENZYME Q10, L-CARNITINE, L-ARGININE, HAWTHORN

Literally found in every cell of the body, **coenzyme Q10,** (Q10) is a vitamin-like substance that is derived from many foods a heart patient *seeks to avoid,* and therein may lie part of the problem. High amounts of Q10 are found in the no-no organ meats kidney and liver, as well as sardines, soybean oil, peanuts and certain fish. A scientist at the *University of Texas at Austin,* Dr. Karl Folkers, discovered the following.

> **Coenzyme Q10 was lacking among heart failure patients. Dr. Folkers determined these same patients showed improvement when the supplement was added to their diets: the heart muscle itself (when subjected to tests) actually showed signs of strengthening.**

Does coenzyme Q10 improve survival rates? Dr. Folkers, along with his study associate Dr. Langsjoen and their team, found encouraging statistics when they evaluated heart failure patients over three years.

**Seventy five percent of those on Q10 therapy along with taking their traditional prescriptions survived. Of those study subjects who had not added the supplement to their medications only 25% remained alive at the end of the study, three years later.**

The successful trials exploring the benefits of Q10 now number in the hundreds, and the conferences devoted to investigating, substantiating and qualifying the positive dramatic affects of coenzyme Q10 are in the record. **Clearly, an improvement was noted when Q10 was taken, with an obvious decline becoming apparent when the supplement had been discontinued among these same subjects.** As has been seen with hypertensive patients, diuretics are prescribed as they become necessary for heart failure patients when pulmonary edema is noted or fluid buildup becomes problematic in the legs. They relieve some of the added work the heart is forced to endure in trying to keep up with adequate heart function and oxygen demands necessary to expel water from the lungs and extremities. One concern facing the patient is that as the tissues are flushed by means of the diuretic, certain critical nutrients are flushed prematurely from the body, and supplementation becomes even more important than normal as it involves *electrolytes* as with the blood pressure medications we read about earlier.

# THE JAPANESE FIRST TO RECOGNIZE

Japan was one of the first to take up the banner for coenzyme Q10 in the 70's, and today more than 6 million people in that country alone use the supplement to combat not only congestive heart failure but also rhythm disturbances and elevated blood pressure. It would almost be assured that if you lived in Japan (or perhaps Italy) and were being treated with conventional medication for heart failure, your doctor would also have you on Q10 as adjunctive therapy. Eight symposia, generating more than 300 papers from the combined work of 200 physicians, agreed that treatment with Q10 improved the heart's pumping action to a significant degree. Also (importantly) there was *no drug interaction noted*. There were no complicated adverse effects recorded other than occasional nausea among a very few patients which could be attributable to Q10 therapy. Earlier trials were conducted by physicians and researchers from a total of 18 separate countries. The largest individual study conducted was the Italian *Baggio* study performed in 1994. This particular study addressed safety, and adjunctive therapy. The enrollment in this study was significant, involving some 2664 heart failure patients.

# COENZYME Q10 FOUND DEFICIENT AMONG HEART FAILURE PATIENTS

The wider medical community in this country is still holding court as to the merits and claims of coenzyme Q10, even though numerous trials have been arriving at the same basic favorable conclusions over the past few years. **Among those conclusions is the fact that blood and tissue levels of Q10 have been found significantly deficient among heart failure patients.** While some cardiomyopathy (enlarged heart) patients were kept on their primary medications, certain of them were administered placebo therapy. A measurement of the *ejection fraction* (which we have discussed earlier) as a means of ultimately determining the strength of the heart's pumping ability was recorded.

## EJECTION FRACTION: UNDENIABLE EVIDENCE

With regard to symptomatic fatigue, palpitations and chest pain, the ejection fraction as a measurement of cardiac output **showed a consistent and sustained improvement among the heart failure patients taking the supplement** compared to those on placebo. *Incredibly, some patients early in their disease, actually* (according to the researchers) *experienced a return to their normal heart size.* A consequence of this dysfunction is its possible contribution to destructive left ventricle enlargement. Sleep apnea patients also are in danger of left ventricle enlargement and should inform their physicians if they become aware of the problem. A 24-hour electrocardiogram halter is often worn to monitor the heart and to record for the doctor how the heart responds during such episodes.

## STATIN DRUGS INHIBIT COENZYME LEVELS

*Here is a shocker. How many doctors are checking their patients' levels of coenzyme while prescribing any of the HMG-CoA reductase inhibitors commonly known as statin drugs? Are you yourself on a cholesterol-lowering statin drug?* One double-blind study led by the "father" of coenzyme Q10, Dr. Karl Folkers, and published in journal *Pharmacology* in 1993, addressed this very question. Folkers found that these drugs (marvelous as they are) did in fact reduce levels of coenzyme Q10 among the patients in a double-blind placebo study. Folkers <u>also</u> had reported three years earlier on a study focusing on the first statin drug, *Lovastatin*. The study results were published in *Proc National Academy of Science* in 1990. The focus was on how levels of Q10 were found reduced in patients prescribed this particular statin. If you are on any statin drug you might do well to discuss this information with your doctor. He or she may be very surprised!

> **In one study, 100 mgs of coenzyme Q10 daily was enough to reverse what had been previously compromised among the patients assigned to various statin therapy.**

## COENZYME Q10 AND CARDIOMYOPATHY

The information from the combined trials dedicated to cardiomyopathy <u>and</u> coenzyme Q10, appeared absolutely outstanding. One such double-blind study reported on the progress or decline of 80 patients over a five-year period. The results claimed **a significant 89% improvement among the participants**. In a separate trial involving 143 subjects the findings were landmark.

## EJECTION FRACTION IMPROVEMENT WAS OBSERVED IN 84% OF THE STUDY PARTICIPANTS

When the study applicants who had been on conventional monolithic therapy were compared to those who were administered *both conventional therapy and the coenzyme supplement, **the group whose regimen included coenzyme Q10 showed an improved survival rate**!* Based on the evidence, what would be the reason not to prescribe heart patients the protection afforded by coenzyme Q10? Confer with your physician, referring him or her to Dr. Folker's findings.

## Q10 AND B6 PRODUCTION DECREASE WITH AGE

There has been recent confirmation that the body's Q10 production and B6 production do decrease with age. Most patients exhibiting symptoms of heart failure are in their senior years, and based on the preceding information, heart failure patients could ill afford a further decline in levels of these two supplements. Coenzyme Q10, as well as B6, is also necessary to favorably affect homocysteine levels. This information concerning the two supplements was a contribution of the work of the *Institute for Biomedical Research*, at the *University of Texas at Austin*, authors Willis R; Anthony M; Sun L; Honse Y; Qiao G.

# WHEN MEDICAL THERAPY FOR HEART FAILURE FAILS, QUALITY OF LIFE AND SURVIVAL WERE IMPROVED WITH COENZYME Q10

The findings of the *Manchester Hospital Study* as reported by Steven T. Sinatra demonstrated an improvement in the patient's **quality of life as well as their rate of survival**. Participants showed both systolic and diastolic function improvement attributable to Q10 therapy. Most important was the finding that coenzyme Q10 had actually produced…

**POSITIVE RESULTS AMONG VERY ADVANCED HEART PATIENTS WHEN ALL PREVIOUS TRADITIONAL MEDICAL THERAPY HAD FAILED.**

**This** is nothing short of revolutionary! **The study recommended that Q10 be included with traditional medicine in adjunctive therapy.** (Source: *Infotrieve*)

## NATURAL TREATMENT FOR CONGESTIVE HEART FAILURE

A clinical research report, published in *Medical Hypotheses* April 96, supported earlier findings and also coined the term "metavitamins." Included in this category along with coenzyme Q10 were *taurine, magnesium, potassium, chromium, L-carnitine and fish oil.* **The report suggested that these supplements, when added to conventional heart**

**failure therapy, provided benefit to congestive heart failure patients.** The conclusion was that since these metavitamins came from nutritional sources, they would (as certain previous studies agreed) carry little or no toxic affect. The report suggested that there was little reason why this benefit from the combination should not be studied as a comprehensive nutritional beneficial therapy for congestive heart failure. As mentioned earlier, CHF is a very serious condition and regardless of the promising claims of researchers and physicians, your own doctor should evaluate the information with you in considering the evidence for combination therapy. Having said this, the information in favor of this supplement is nothing short of miraculous.

## 53.6% QUALITY OF LIFE IMPROVEMENT

Under the same heading of improvement to the **quality of life,** consider the report from the Department of Internal Medicine, from *Buaai Hospital,* Reggio Emilia in 1994, After enrolling some 2664 test subjects in a cross section of 173 centers in Italy, positive improvement in *three symptoms* that are normally associated with heart failure were found. The study reported an overall improvement in the **quality of life witnessed by 53.6% of those patients in the study**. The dosages administered ranged from 50-150 mgs of Q10 daily.

## ADDITIONAL BENEFIT

A study from the *Department of Physiology* at the *University of Granada,* Spain, suggested that this supplement *can offer a protective effect in warding off the damage of oxidation and free radical attack against cellular aging by enriching the membranes with monounsaturated fatty acids.*

## WORTHY OPPONENTS CONVINCED

The study authors from the *Department of Cardiology, Aalborg Hospital* in Denmark, the team of Munkholm H; Hansen HH; and Rasmussen K, embarked on an invasive study to confirm or debunk previous non-invasive studies that had made positive claims about the effectiveness of this particular supplement.

## ABSOLUTELY AMAZING
## COENZYME Q10 RESULTS!

The researchers implemented a 3-minute stress test followed by an invasive right heart catherization among patients who had demonstrated a very low initial (left ventricle) ejection fraction of 26%!

---

**The researchers found after 12 weeks of therapy that those subjects in the double-blind trial receiving 100 mgs of Q10 twice daily HAD SHOWN SIGNIFICANT LEFT VENTRICLE IMPROVEMENT.**

---

They further confirmed that the stroke index and pulmonary artery pressure also improved among treated patients. Congestive heart failure patients would benefit from an adjunctive treatment with coenzyme Q10.

# L-CARNITINE

Produced by the amino acids *lysine* and *methionine,* **car-nitine** has been shown in studies to help in the treatment of CHF by minimizing the destruction that this ailment inflicts on heart muscle.

> **Congestive heart failure patients have repeatedly shown in studies to be deficient in adequate amounts of *L-Carnitine*.**

This deficiency manifests itself when damage is created by a lack of oxygenation of the membranes and heart muscle. Unfortunately, this is not a problem unique to HF patients. Incidentally, *L-Carnitine* is not one of the essential amino acids and, consequently, must be supplemented.

# HAWTHORN
# (CRATAEGUS OXYACANTHA)

Pharmaceutical companies in this country for more than twenty years invested heavily in an effort to discover a drug that could increase a patient's cardiac output—a drug that could actually enhance the **beating function** of the heart. A weakened heart (whether by myocardial infarction or subsequent heart failure) loses its ability to pump adequately, which eventually results in heart damage and general decline. The new experimental class of drugs was called *Inotrope* drugs. They initially showed great promise and received much attention from the cardiovascular industry at large. According to Keith Aaronson,

M.D., in an article entitled *"Hawthorn for the heart"* which appeared in several publications including *Heart Watch* explained, all the Inotrope drugs that were under study at the time had "actually raised" the death rate in people with heart failure. According to Aaronson's explanation, they probably did so by helping to cause fatal rhythm disturbances in the heart's main pumping chambers (the ventricles). The one exception to the experimental drugs (as reported) was a drug currently being prescribed named digoxin or lanoxin. In the meantime, they might have all saved their money. An herb known as *hawthorn*, a derivative of the *hawthorn berry*, has been successfully prescribed as adjunct heart therapy for decades throughout Europe and in other parts of the world. Hawthorn has shown almost zero recorded negative complications. So effective have been the claims attributed to the herb over the decades that the national drug investigation bureau in Germany gave approval for *hawthorn* to be <u>sold</u> as a drug. Like aspirin, *hawthorn* has numerous benefits for cardiovascular health. Not only does it **enhance the pumping action of the heart**, it also encourages the natural *heart rhythm*, providing a degree of intervention in preventing *arrhythmias*. We addressed *arterial spasms* in an earlier chapter, and *hawthorn* is believed to interfere positively with this dangerous dysfunction. Simultaneously hawthorn inhibits certain of the blood clotting factors in its offering of prostaglandins.

**There are other documented claims that the heart muscle itself is strengthened by this herb, which even lowers blood pressure and diminishes angina pain.**

The benefits attributed to this herb as an adjunct treatment for heart patients is legendary and has been so for decades.

*Hawthorn has been shown to increase the actual pumping contractions of the heart.*

It increases not only the blood flow from the heart, but the distribution throughout the body including distribution to the extremities.

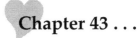

# Chapter 43

# SUPPLEMENTS *(cont'd)*
## *L-Arginine and Nitric Oxide, Taurine, Bilberry*

### NOBEL PRIZE AWARDED

To warrant such a prestigious acknowledgement, the role of *nitric oxide* as a signaling molecule in the cardiovascular system was obviously an important discovery. The prize was handed to Louis J. Ignarro and his team in the *Molecular and Medical Parmacology Department* at *UCLA*. Endothelial damage, as we have discussed, occurs to the cells and linings of the arterial wall following a series of assaults, including a destructive companionship with free radicals and subsequent oxidation. These and other injurious factors take their toll in reducing the artery's ability to *vasodilate* in response to the body's needs. A non-essential amino acid (one not produced by our bodies), *L-arginine, may be the best source **available for the production of nitric oxide**.*

Studies have shown oral administration of L-arginine to be a helpful mediator in diminishing endothelial dysfunction and damage (journal *Clinical Pharmacology Ther.* 2001). Many people are taking the controversial Human Growth Hormone by injection at a cost of approximately $28K per year. Others ingest the peptide in capsule form to stimulate the pituitary gland's declining production of HGH in the aging process. **Interestingly,** a natural source of HGH production is the combination of L-*arginine/L-orithine.* The amino acid in this combination also extends benefit to the patient experiencing "hardening of the arteries." It therefore affords a double bonus for heart patients as well as those wishing to receive the hormone's youthful benefit. This approach may not be as immediately effective as shots, but is probably a lot safer. *We are, however, specifically addressing cardiovascular disease and arginine's ability to produce nitric oxide, which has a definitive, positive role in both venous and arterial health, according to the research.*

## OXIDATION, FREE RADICALS AND LDL

Oxidation damages arteries. There are people with normal LDL cholesterol who still have a significant degree of *free radical oxidative* forces working destructively in their systems. The level of LDL alone cannot be a full predictor of risk. In contrast, another patient might present with very high LDLC but with little or no atherosclerosis. Studies have shown that such fortunate patients experience less atheroclerosis simply because of a low degree of free radical oxidative activity. Smoking, lack of exercise and inadequate antioxidant intake are all elements that create arterial damage. There has been a lot of press about the health advantages attributed to blueberries as a mediator against oxidation. A *University of California* study has found that blueberries do specifically inhibit LDL oxidation. Bananas, grape seed extract, pycnogenol, alpha lipoic acid and vitamins A, E and C are natural allies in this fight, along with arginine.

## ADITIONAL BENEFITS FROM L-ARGININE

According to RH Boger, Bode-Boger SM of the *Institute of Clinical Pharmocology, Hannover Medical School,* Hannover, Germany, *L-Arginine is the precursor of nitric oxide* and has been shown to improve endothelial function in animal tests upon <u>immediate prescription</u>. *According to the report, this amino acid has also been shown to improve the very important endothelium-dependent vasodilation in both hyper-cholesterol patients and those with atherosclerosis.* A number of long-term studies have concluded that *oral administration of L-arginine* can improve clinical symptoms of cardiovascular disease in humans.

## TAURINE

Taurine, another of the amino acids, is involved with the nervous system, but also affects the muscle system, and therein lies the reason **taurine has been used for the treatment of congestive heart failure.** Heart failure is a condition that destroys the heart muscle, diminishing the heart's ability to pump. The belief is that *taurine may be helpful in controlling the patient's actual heartbeat.*

## BILBERRY

More and more articles are in the news exalting the outstanding antioxidant health benefits of blueberries. Blueberries are American as blueberry pie while in Europe the variety, the cousin, is the bilberry. It is a powerful *flavonoid* producer and reported to contain 10-15 times greater antioxidant properties than vitamin C. One study concluded bilberry was 50 times more effective as an antioxidant than even vitamin E. Flavonoids besides their antioxidant qualities also serve in removing metals from the system. Bilberry for the cardiovascular patient offers another weapon against oxidation but also helps maintain proper blood pressure and is involved in inhibiting the blood clotting aggregation process. Bilberry also strengthens capillary walls and extends its benefits to help protect arterial flexibility. This herb has been used in Europe for decades for both arterial health as well as treatment of certain eye disorders.

## ON THE HORIZON FOR CHF PATIENTS?

Good news travels fast, and many drugs are in development to aid in treating this killer. This characterization of heart failure is accurate because **half the people who have the advanced stage of this illness will not survive a full year, according to the clinical evidence.** What makes this a particularly exciting time is the fact that although not much encouraging news has been coming from the pharmaceutical companies over the past 10-20 years with regard to better medications for heart failure, hopefully that will soon change.

# Chapter 44

# IMPLANTABLE *mechanical*
# PACEMAKERS

E nter this life-saving device. This remark-able invention has been around for decades and has provided salvation for thousands. Its purpose is to provide a mechanical substitute for a failed or failing *natural pacemaker* within someone's body. Complications arose in the early models when they were introduced. Any new mechanical invention (in-cluding the mechanical heart currently in early

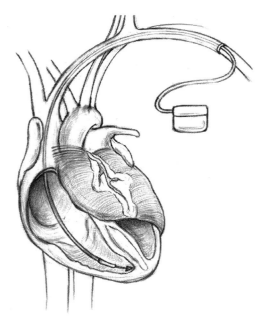

**Fig 7: Pacemaker**

stages of application) will have its share of failures along the road to final acceptance. While today's types have battery lives of 6+ years, the earlier models had poor battery reliability and relatively higher mechanical failure rates. Newer generations of the pacemaker have all but eliminated these problems. One complication of the earlier devices was that they too often malfunctioned over-compensating in their appointed task in attempting to correct a failing heartbeat. Instead of stabilizing *brady-cardia*, (a slow heartbeat) these malfunctioning units could actually set the heart beating frantically in the opposite direction creating the condition known as *traycardyia (very fast heartbeat)*. Your physician or cardiologist, in assessing your individual profile, might ask if you experience symptoms such as lightheadedness, dizziness, extreme or unusual fatigue, fainting spells or shortness of breath. It is important that you accurately recall if you have experienced such events in order for your doctor to accurately assess your condition. This would not be a time for denial. Too many macho patients, for instance, shrug off reporting such indications. "No, I haven't felt better in my life." Your doctor listens to you with a keen ear, and what may seem trivial to you in the totality of the examination may help him or her a great deal in helping you avoid a future cardiovascular or stroke event.

## THE DEMAND PACEMAKER

In the case of certain forms of bradycardia, implantable pacemakers are a very necessary and permanent welcomed aid. This type of pacemaker is programmed and activates to compensate for a heartbeat that drops to 60. The unit begins its rescue by bringing the heart rate to a normal level. This type of pacemaker is called a *demand pacemaker* and simply responds and adjusts to the demands that would normally be required of a healthy heart. Before a patient leaves the hospital after implantation, adjustments and necessary compensations are made for that particular individual's needs. This remarkable instrument currently works in cooperation with more than 475,000 American hearts. Anyone who is in need of this technology should welcome it in all of its advanced technological glory. On the horizon are newer variations with capabilities beyond what is now available. There are ongoing studies working towards the development of a pacemaker designed for heart failure, the rapidly growing health problem we have addressed as presenting a particular crisis in the aging population. This device is being designed to better facilitate *Biventricular pacing*, in directing its technological strength at stimulating and aiding both the left and right ventricles in their appointed task by coordinating the distribution of blood. **A person with weakened ventricle function may in the foreseeable future receive the benefit of this advancement in pacemaker technology.** Today many devices are advanced to the point that they use incredible intelligent technology to literally shock the heart back into correct rhythm if required. It is a similar function as when a physician applies the paddles to a patient's failed heart in a hospital emergency. These pacemakers often intervene in preventing what could be an episodic brush with sudden death. They are a life-saving advancement.

## THE NEW TECHNOLOGY

The recent versions can actually function at various output levels in **accordance with the patient's individual needs.** As the body calls for higher output as it would in a case of heightened physical activity or emotional stress, the pacemaker functions accordingly to meet the increased demands. The newer versions also have much improved *fail-safe* capability and reliability.

## A PACER FOR ATRIAL FIBRILLATION

*Atrial fibrillation* remains a constant threat to the life of anyone with heart disease, and, yes, another next-generation pacemaker is being developed for this condition. The technology is called *atrial pacing*. This promising advancement will actually move to action in the event that the upper left and right atrium begin to spasm, a condition too often fatal.

## TACHYCARDIA
### *(Fast Heartbeat)*

With *tachycardia,* the heart beats faster than 100 beats per minute continually or for prolonged periods. It is the direct opposite condition of *bradycardia* (slow heartbeat). A pacemaker can be programmed to slow the beat to a normal rhythm (between 60 and 100 beats per minute). This pacemaker functions very much like a "governor" in an automobile's mechanical engine that only permits the car's speed or RPM to reach certain thresholds. Patients who are wearing implanted pacemakers are cautioned by their various manufacturers to avoid a close or extended proximity to microwaves, certain powerful radio transmitters, electric shavers and, certainly, security detection systems one might encounter at airports. In reality, the very brief time one might be exposed walking by such a device is so transient that manufacturers do not believe there is much of a threat. They do not however, advise tarrying at these spots for long periods of time. The whole world has gone cell phone crazy, and there has been some speculation about the dangers to those cell phone users wearing implantable devices. The advice seems to be, refrain from "pocketing" an activated cell phone directly over the heart area. One suggestion offered is to hold the cell phone to the opposite ear from your pacemaker as an added precaution. It makes sense.

I have used the terms "heart attack" (MI) and "stroke" many, many times in this book, however, the word "clot" as in "blood clot" appears almost twice as many times as the other two terms.

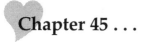 Chapter 45 . . .

# CLOTS

## cause *of* 89-90%
## *of heart and stroke attacks*

One might wonder if enough attention is directed at what could be done diagnostically to discover and inhibit the ultimate cause of heart attack and stroke. In other words, is there enough focus directed at preempting the formation of a clot?

**IS IT NOT THE CLOT THAT ACTUALLY CAUSES THE HEART ATTACK? IS IT NOT THE CLOT THAT IN THE FINAL ANALYSIS LODGES IN THE BRAIN INITIATING A STROKE, OR TRAVELS TO THE LUNGS AND THE PULMONARY ARTERY?**

The three mechanisms of stroke are *embolism* (which reaches the brain via arterial route), *thrombosis* (from a formation of a *thrombus* which occurs at the wall of the artery), and thirdly, the *hemorrhagic* result when a blood vessel ruptures. Uncontrolled hypertension can also be the cause of this third access. According to the American Medical Encyclopedia, between 40 and 50% of strokes can be attributed to thrombosis, another 30-35% to embolism and the remaining 20-25% to hemorrhages in one of two forms, *intracerebral* (inside the brain itself) and *subarachnoid* (occurring on the exterior surface). There are also small clots that gather on the leaflets of a *mitral* or *aortic* valve and pose an ever-present risk of dislodgment.

## THE CLOT, THE CLOT, THE CLOT!

Aspirin (ASA) is of major importance in averting heart attack, but aspirin alone cannot offer all the protection a particular blood chemistry might require. There are approximately 11 additional pathways in which blood clots can form, and aspirin, though it does interfere with platelet aggregation, will not sufficiently block all of the other receptors. When one experiences either an MI or stroke, immediate steps are taken to thin and monitor the blood to try to ensure that the event will not be repeated.

## THINKING OUTSIDE THE BOX

Hypercoagulation and hyperplatelet aggregation are the two major pathways leading to MI or stroke. There are now various drugs to interfere with each of these two pathways. The problem is none of these drugs would be administered preventively unless the physician had done the necessary tests to identify those at risk. This advanced testing is not part of the customary approach mandated by current protocol or insurance guidelines. The routine blood tests including the INR would not necessarily reveal one's propensity toward clot formation until it was learned much too late, after an event had taken place.

It would be more productive from a preventive standpoint to concentrate more on these factors and receptors by monitoring more closely the very things that would actually permit the small, apparently insignificant clot to collect and eventually manifest as the major, "killer" clot. Dr. Julian Whitaker, physician/author and founder of the *Whitaker Wellness Center*, personally takes two capsules of cayenne pepper daily to inhibit or break down the formation of tiny clots. The question of whether or not enough attention is paid to clotting factors probably answers itself when one looks at the 600,000 strokes a year happening to Americans, and the more than a million heart attacks. Add to these numbers the newest findings released, that 11 million people yearly are suffering "silent strokes." There is obviously more diagnostic effort needed if common sense and imagination were the criteria of final decision. It was Albert Einstein who once said, "*Imagination is more important than knowledge.*" Well Albert, if we permitted ourselves to imagine a fair and equitable way to cut the costs of expensive prescription medications in this country what would you think of this possible solution? It is a fact; pharmaceutical companies spend millions to bring a drug through the trial process to market. It is also true they have a limited 7 year period of time in which to realize their profit before the drug qualifies for generic distribution. The company's costs appear justified inasmuch as many millions of dollars are lost on the developmental highway as drugs fall out of favor along the approval road. While their argument is sound, there might be a compromised solution that would treat both private industry and the patient more fairly. **I have not** heard anyone suggest that the government might simply increase the patent protection from 7 years to 14 years with the caveat that the companies would have to agree to cut the cost to the public in half. Might this provide common ground for agreement? Would this be too simple a solution to a monumental problem, Albert?

## NORTHWICK PARK STUDY

In the *Northwick Park Study* a direct relationship was confirmed between the thrombogenic state of a patient and cardiovascular artery disease. The following on-point study addressed only two clotting factors, but the information is pertinent to the subject at hand. It appeared in the *European Heart Journal*, offered by P.M. Sweetnam, H. Thomas, and J. Yarnell. The study objective was to report on the ten-year follow-up of the *Caerphilly and Speedwell* studies. These studies' concentration was on how fibrinogen and viscosity (blood thickness) would contribute to the prediction of incidence of *ischemic* heart disease. After all other risk factors were taken into account, and both fibrinogen and viscosity were added to the risk profile, they jointly served as predictors of an increase in *ischemic* heart disease. *It did not matter which of the two markers increased,* whether it was fibrinogen or viscosity. If either of the two levels became elevated, the risk was increased. The abstract concluded...

*" Fibrinogen and viscosity are powerful, long-term and independent predictors of the risk of ischemic heart disease. "*

## PATHOLOGICAL FACTORS

This area involves mechanisms that are generated by *pathological* factors at the vessel wall. Among the tests seldom given to determine more advanced causes for blood clotting are: *Plasminogen activator inhibitor, (PAI-1), interluken 6, tissue plasminogen activator, (t-Pa), D-dimmer of fibrin, glycoprotein IIa/IIIb, hematocrit, hemoglobin, Von Willebrand factor VII and homocysteine.* All influence the way your body is handling clotting issues. If you have advancing heart or stroke disease and would like to have the benefit of these tests, talk to your doctor about paying the difference if your insurance won't cover them. These tests are not the run-of-the-mill evaluations.

## AN AUTHOR'S JOURNEY
## (PART TWO CONTINUED)
### *Searching for the Causes*

Finally, in my early journey I was fortunate to meet Dr. Mark Bell, M.D., an open-minded progressive physician, who owns and operates E.R. and emergency family clinics in southern California who would be the first doctor of those I had consulted who did not think the direction I was exploring in late 1997 was without merit. Tests I was requesting for inflammation, opportune infections and inherited risk factors made perfectly good sense to him even though they were not mainstream. My blood was drawn and sent express mail to the *Berkeley Heartlab* for inherited factors and an electrophoresis LDL study. The immediate results showed a relatively strong type "B" classification (a factor you have read about earlier in the book). What was especially interesting was that even though I had already been taking 800 mcgs of folic acid each day for the prior six months (twice the general recommendation), my homocysteine test score was still, in spite of the 800 mcgs of folic acid, 8.7. Not that this score was alarming but from a research standpoint one could only speculate what the level of homocysteine must have been during the prior 15-20 years of my *life without the benefit of 800 mcgs of folic acid.* Of course this would remain an unanswered question. A range of 13-15 or higher would have certainly been possible. Given my protracted earlier history of highly elevated fibrinogen, we decided to test again by evaluating Factor VII. Factor VII and Factor I are markers that determine the level of fibrinogen in a patient's blood. It was still significantly higher than acceptable.

## THE COLLECTIVE TEST RESULTS

▶ LDL subfractions study (electrophoresis) determined an undesirable type "B"
▶ Homocysteine score (which would later prove to be an important factor) was *at this* time 8.7
▶ Lp (a), inherited gene, an ideal score of 1
▶ Fibrinogen, extremely elevated

**Inflammatory test results** for,

▶ C. pneumoniae infection (positive)
▶ Epstein barr infection (positive)
▶ Helicobacter Pylori (negative)
▶ C-reactive protein (negative)

# TREATMENT

▶ Apolipoprotein "B" treated with niacin
▶ Chlamydia pneumonaie with *Zithromax*
▶ Epstein barr (not treated)

*Antiphospholipin antibody syndrome* (APL), a serious blood clotting disorder, was found by accident when the lab misunderstood an order for a IIb/IIIa glycoprotein test and in error substituted a similar sounding but very different beta 2 glycoprotein test. The error resulted in a positive identification of another inherited silent risk factor. APL affects the clotting process and is a contributing cause of stroke. With two major clotting factors *fibrinogen* and *APL* now identified, it would be even more imperative to closely monitor clotting factors. Ordering these sophisticated tests proved to be an important step in controlling and avoiding future consequence.

# TUNNEL VISION

If a physician or assistant looks quickly at the CBC blood work chart following your office visit, they may simply be glancing to see if anything is marked "out of range." Often times a nurse may scan the results and call attention to the doctor if something jumps off the scale. Here is how *tunnel vision* can cause an individual to miss the very factors that can cause a heart attack or stroke. If a combination of viscosity aggregation or coagulating factors are at the top of the scale but are short of actually being out of range, what would be the proper interpretation?

# CREATIVE THINKING

*Let's consider the following as an example:* A patient's hematocrit (viscosity) score is one point down from the top of the reference scale and his or her hemoglobin score is right near the top. Both are arguably within range and probably would not alert most physicians to a problem. However, these two seemingly innocent scores, in combination, along with an unrealized elevated fibrinogen or homocysteine or CRP level, may together be setting a lethal appointment for a major heart attack or stroke. Does this make the point that certain catastrophes might escape detection under the current protocols? Preventive medicine does not always adhere to the normally accepted ranges that have been in general use for the past forty years. On those scales, the borderline scores would be way out of whack! Standards do get changed, as did cholesterol and triglyceride guidelines within the past two years. On page 343 are the currently accepted reference range standards and the optimal recommendations as suggested by the *Life Extension Foundation.*

## SUMMARY

You are now aware of some of the ways blood clots can form, leading to eventual crisis. The pathways are created through viscosity (thickness), hypercoagulation (over tendency to coagulate), hyperaggregation (clumping of platelets), and physiological (physical destructive factors) originating at the artery wall itself. We have also discussed a battery of sophisticated but less known blood tests a physician may use when someone is thought to be at risk. These tests can provide very critical evidence of what might be happening

with regard to pending attacks in time to identify and
mediate the specific source of the clot's formation before
an attack takes place. The object, obviously, is to prevent
the preventable. An ounce of prevention...

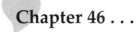

# Chapter 46

# *Life Extension's*
# OPTIMAL RANGE SCALE

| BLOOD TEST | STANDARD | OPTIMAL |
|---|---|---|
| Fibrinogen | 460 | under 300 mg/dl |
| C-reactive protein | up to 4.9 mg/l | under 2mg/L |
| Homocysteine | up to 15 micro mol/L | under 7 |
| Glucose | up to 109 mg/dl | under 100 mg/dl |
| Iron | up to 180 mg/dl | under 100 mcg/dl |
| Cholesterol | up to 199 mg/dl | between 180-220 mg/dl |
| LDL C | up to 129 mg/dl | under 100 mg/dl |
| HDL C | no lower than 35 | over 50 mg/dl |
| Triglycerides | up to 199 mg/dl | under 100 mg/dl |

The preceding appears by expressed permission of the *Life Extension Foundation*, a health organization that has consistently been ahead of the curve.

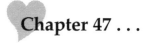

Chapter 47 . . .

# *IRON*

We were told some years ago that if a man gave blood once or twice a year through a blood bank, like the Red Cross, they would reduce their risk of heart attack by a significant percentage. At the same time they would be helping someone who might need blood for actual survival.

## 88% REDUCED RISK AMONG
## BLOOD DONORS

This dramatic statistic which appeared in a 1998 issue of the *American Journal of Epidemiology* should get one's attention. If you will forgive the comparison; as healthy as it is for the life of an automobile engine to have its oil drained, it is apparently also healthy to remove a pint of blood once or twice a year from one's body. Why then does the Red Cross have a continual shortage of blood supply? Is it due to more fear of the needle than the heart attack? Eighty-eight percent less risk should be a real motivator. There is another theory that has been put forward and that is part of the reduced risk may be coming from the fact that oxidized cholesterol is also removed in the process, which may be lowering the heart disease risk in general.

There have been as many as 24 studies done under various criteria to determine if in fact excessive *ferritin* (iron) is a risk factor for heart disease and heart attack. Several of these studies have produced conflicting reports on iron's involvement. Supplements or iron-rich food are needed in a younger women's physiology because of the amount of iron she expels through the monthly menstrual cycle. Pregnant women naturally require higher iron intake than would young menstrual women. Replenishment is therefore required to tip the balance in the woman's favor. There is a difference in the role iron plays in a man's diet compared to what is required by menstrual women. The problem is compounded when men who do not have a route for expending or eliminating iron unwittingly take supplements or multi-vitamins that provide additional iron. As well, men on heavy meat diets might want to pay particular attention to their iron levels. (Incidentally, vitamin manufacturers have paid heed to these findings, and now eliminate or diminish the amount of iron added in the preparation of men's multi-vitamins). On the other side of the issue, it has been suggested that endurance athletes and dedicated vegetarians might be less able to maintain iron levels, and may find it necessary to augment their iron intake to meet daily requirements. Two familiar *iron*-rich food sources are raisins and liver.

The *Rotterdam Study* addressing *"Serum Ferritin and Risk of Myocardial Infarction in the Elderly"* reported on a study authored by Dr. D. Trichopoulos of the *Harvard School of Public Health* from the *University of Athens, Greece* and *Na-*

*tional School of Public Health.* The study conclusions were: *With each 50 mg monthly increase of iron intake the risk of heart disease for senior men and women grew 1.4 times, (140%). Women over 60 (according to the study) were 3.5 times (350%) as likely to have heart disease for the same 50 mg amount of monthly increase in ferritin score.*

> **Both men and women over age 60 and men who have had a high intake of iron were at greater risk for heart disease.**

## "IRON GENE" MUTATION IDENTIFIED

In September of 1999, two separate research teams made public their findings supporting the earlier studies and claims, that too much iron can in fact increase the number of heart attacks. **More specifically, both teams identified a gene mutation that is believed responsible for confounding the body's ability to process iron normally. The research suggests that this condition definitely increases one's chances of having a heart attack and** risk of one's dying of heart disease. There are two copies of this gene, called the **HFE gene,** which determine how the body will regulate and store iron. If both of these gene copies are defective, a condition called *hemochromatosis can exist.* This ailment permits an unnaturally high level of iron to accumulate in the body. *Hereditary Hemochromatosis* **(HH) affects 1 in 300-400 people (significant odds) and has been said to be the most commonly inherited of the genetic disorders.** The end result of HH can be the malfunction or dysfunction of bodily organs, which include the *heart, liver and pancreas.*

There are two things being discussed here:

► High amounts of ferritin are not advisable for men in general, and losing some iron through blood donations adds to one's chances of avoiding a heart attack.

► There is now an identified HFE inherited iron gene mutation that can play a role in heart attack.

Notwithstanding, newly introduced clinical study results, by Dr. Romi-Pekka Tuomainen from the *University of Kuopio, Finland* informed that; among the 1,150 men in the study, **77 (6.7%) were identified as carriers of the HFE *mutated* Tyr 282 iron gene.** According to the report, "Male carriers of the common *hemochromatosis* gene mutation are at a 2-fold risk for first (heart attack) compared with non-carriers." For each 100 microgram of ferritin elevation in the group with the abnormal gene, their risk of heart attack increased by 25%. The researchers believe these subjects would benefit from treatment to reduce the amount of iron stored within their blood streams. The only way to eliminate high stores is to bleed, and giving blood is still the only way.

## AN INHERITED DEFECTIVE IRON GENE

In 1981 Dr. Sullivan, who first put forth what has been called the *"iron hypothesis"* as a risk for cardiovascular disease, reported to Reuter's, "But if this is true [iron stores being a risk factor] **then small increases in stored iron are a risk factor for myocardial infarction."** Dr. Jerome Sullivan, from the *University of Florida* in Gainesville, claimed "carriers" are a large part of the population. **He speculates 10 to 30% of people may carry at least one defective gene for *hemochromatosis.*** This according to the news article excerpted from Dr. Sullivan's presentation.

" **Carriers almost always don't know they are at increased risk. They have almost no increase in iron stores, but that small increase is significant and that small increase is probably what caused the increased incidence (of heart disease deaths).** "

How concerned should one be? Could something as seemingly inconsequential as a slight elevation in ferritin value have this much importance and affect on human life, as the research indicates? Dr. Sullivan offered, that the "iron hypothesis" explains why young, menstruating women have a very low risk of cardiovascular disease and death. He added that these values fall in the range of 20-40 mg/dl. A level *below* 20 presents reason for your doctor's concern as well as values *over* 80. Remember the *iron deficiency anemia* commercials for "Tired Blood" many years ago? The cure was to take a certain iron-rich tonic. The commercials left the impression that the more iron supplement one took the better they would feel. What was that all about? There is, to be sure, such an ailment, and it is the most common form of anemia, but were listeners being given indiscriminate blanket advice? The following short list is food sources that provide necessary iron: chicken, turkey, eggs, red meat, fish, peas, beans, fortified cereals and enriched breads.

# RED MEAT THE MAIN CULPRIT

To be fair there is still some controversy regarding the actual role ferritin plays in heart disease. The studies, regardless of their final conclusions, agree universally on one thing: RED MEAT is the most acknowledged source of high levels of iron.

## TOO LITTLE IRON!

On the other end of the spectrum is the exact opposite problem of having *very low iron*. The issue here is one of anemia, *too little iron,* and the discovery of a gene that inhibits the necessary absorption of iron by the body. Dr. Andrew T. McKie, associated with *King's College* in the UK, searched the genetic database and found the responsible gene. According to McKie, with chronic anemia the amount of Dcytb protein produced by this defective gene elevates as the body unsuccessfully fights to restore normal levels of iron. People who are anemic may have symptoms of dizziness, headache, shortness of breath and predominant fatigue. Other symptoms may include memory dysfunction, achy joints, heart palpitations and in some cases jaundice indicated by (yellow pallor). These very symptoms may also be present in several other illnesses. The presence of dark stool may correlate with low iron stores and anemia, but these same symptoms may as well indicate the source of the bleeding is from an ulcer or a vital organ. These are all symptoms that require a doctor's determination as to the actual cause.

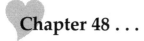

# Chapter 48

*The Oscar goes to the*

# BEST DRUG

## *in 100 years...*

Aspirin celebrated its 100th birthday at the beginning of the new century, and what a history.

> A C-reactive protein study following subjects over an eight-year period concluded that those taking aspirin had a reduction of heart attack risk of 55.7%.

Newer, additional uses for aspirin in health therapy are still being explored. At the time of this writing, trials are going on around the world for aspirin's involvement in treating several diseases and conditions, among them Alzheimer's. An earlier study, performed in 1995 at *Johns Hopkins Alzheimer's Disease Research Center*, found encouraging results for many patients whose speech and orientation skills improved by aspirin therapy. Other studies confirm aspirin may also have a role in delaying senility and even in preventing cataracts. Most recently, a study involving women explored the possibility that aspirin can also reduce the number of ovarian cancer cases. In one trial it was documented those who used aspirin as part of their regular regimen reduced their risk of dying of colorectal cancer by as much as 50% compared to non-aspirin users. The drug (according to *Bayer*) was developed more than a 100 years ago in 1897 by a chemist named Felix Hoffmann. Research has revealed however, that *Hippocrates* was prescribing willow bark for relief of pain as far back as 400 years before Christ. Willow bark, contains *salicylic acid*. This acid is precisely the important ingredient found in your tiny little "miracle" aspirin. Wouldn't you know it— Hippocrates never even applied for a patent! Around 1920, people started using aspirin for treating lumbago, nerve pain and rheumatism. A doctor, Lawrence Craven, in 1948 first subscribed to the theory that this drug might provide a benefit for patients in reducing heart attack. **It would take another 32 years before the FDA approved aspirin for treatment and risk reduction of stroke in the event an individual experienced a "mini-stroke" sometimes referred to as a TIA.** Translated, the medical description is *transient ischemic attack*. Treatment probably was advised for these patients because anything that could aid in dissolving the clot or increasing blood flow at this critical time is welcomed therapy. When someone experiences a mini-stroke it is often a precursor to an impending major stroke. The risk is great, and anything that can ward off such a threat would be an effort worth taking even if there is small calculated risk involved. Incidentally, the following symptoms, should you or someone you know ever experience them could be a warning of a TIA in progress: a temporary blackout, with the patient regaining consciousness but awakening disoriented, possibly not knowing where they are or even what day it is; slurred speech and/

or difficulty in focusing; blurred vision, possibly affecting only one eye may also be a post-episodic symptom. These are transient symptoms, and the patient recovering might tend to slough off the actual import of the incident. The patient should realize that it might be the warning of bigger things to come and seek immediate medical attention. Carotid stenosis (in the neck arteries) is definitely something the doctor will evaluate. Ever wonder why doctors put a stethoscope to the patient's neck during a physical? Well, they aren't listening for the seashore. The physician will be able to hear advancing occlusion in the carotid artery. To determine the extent of the stenosis, a (non-invasive) doppler ultrasound evaluation may be ordered if there is concern.

## ASPIRIN AND OVARIAN CANCER

Of the 14,000 women enrolled and studied in the *New York University Women's Health Study* the following results were recorded and reported by the study's lead author, Associate Professor *Arsian Akhmedkhanov,* M.D..

> **Upon a 12 year follow up period, the findings were that women who took aspirin three or more times a week showed a reduction in their risk of becoming positive for ovarian cancer by a significant 40%.**

The reason given by the study author for the reduction of ovarian cancer cases was due to a reduction in chronic inflammation. There is even evidence that this wonder drug may help deter certain forms of cancer by inhibiting the cancer cells' ability to attach themselves to tissue walls.

# ON THE DOWNSIDE, REYES SYNDROME

On the negative side of the coin, warnings were issued in 1988 by the *Federal Drug Association* cautioning parents not to use the drug for children because of the risk of developing *Reyes* disease. The same organization soon added that pregnant women should refrain from aspirin therapy during the last three months of their pregnancies. **Finally, as late as 1996, the *FDA* approved aspirin for application during an actual heart attack in progress,** forty-eight years after Dr. Lawrence Cravens first began using it as a protective against heart attack. Here is just one more example of how advanced research is often far ahead of mainstream medicine. Personally, I began taking a daily aspirin in 1979 after becoming aware of the physician trial in progress. I was not about to wait 15 years.

*Dr. Charles Hennekens,* is a professor at the *Boston, Harvard Medical School* and lead author of a report, investigated the advantage of taking aspirin at the first signs of a heart attack. In the study (involving some 17,000 men and women) it was found that patients with the symptoms of a heart attack were less likely to die or have a subsequent heart attack if they had taken a 162 milligram aspirin within 24 hours prior to the onset of symptoms. The study also indicated that patients do not know to turn to aspirin at the first signs of an attack. It had been suggested by *Dr. Hennekens* that one should, at the first sign of a heart attack, take a 325 mg. tablet of aspirin. (He defined the outset symptoms of an attack as crushing chest pain that radiates into the jaw, arm or back.)

"Despite its clear benefits in this clinical setting, aspirin as a treatment for acute myocardial infarction remains underused." The report goes on to say that only 61% of medical patients had been taking aspirin within two days of a hospitalization for heart attack, and a 1993 survey of 1000 hospitals found that just 77% of acute heart attack patients received aspirin therapy.

## STILL AND ALL, THERE IS A RISK

If you have ever wondered what the active ingredient in the aspirin compound is...it is acetylsalicylic acid (ASA). A *Bayer* spokesman believes the little pill could save an additional 100,000 lives a year if more people were taking it regularly. Of course, one would expect the *Bayer* spokesman to be somewhat bias. It is, however, truer than fiction. How many people through the years didn't know the benefit they were deriving when they took an aspirin for a headache and unknowingly prevented a heart attack or stroke? Imagine all the heart attacks this tiny pill must have prevented, and those heart attacks and strokes where it had minimized the damage. It is even recommended to pop one in someone's mouth who is actually exhibiting the symptoms of a heart attack. Remember the *commercials* the company used several years ago? "In just 30 minutes Bayer aspirin is ready to go to work." In 1990, I rode in the ambulance with a dear friend who had just had a serious stroke. When we arrived at the hospital he was given a CT scan and I was present when the doctor evaluated the results. While his gaze was still fixed on the X-ray I asked the doctor, "on a scale of one to ten how would you rate the damage?" He said an 8½ and then asked, "has this man been taking aspirin?" I told him he had stopped taking it about four weeks earlier. The doctor speculated that had he continued the aspirin he probably would have avoided this stroke.

## WHY ASPIRIN DOES NOT ALWAYS STOP HEART ATTACKS AND STROKE

It would be helpful, at this point, to understand the principle that governs platelet aggregation. To put it simply, the problem facing the researchers was finding a drug to circumvent the condition of *platelet clumping* that permits the platelets to stick together in the formation of a clot. The result is called a thrombus (as in thrombosis). It was the hope of researchers under the leadership of study author Dr. Juana Valles, from the *University Hospital La Fe,* in Valencia Spain, that by blocking the substance *thromboxane,* the clotting of the platelets would become a non-event. The problem was that some patients, 45% of those in the trial, still continued to aggregate or bind platelets together with red blood cells even with less *thromboxane.* The objective sought was to <u>prevent</u> the "sticking" of the platelets entirely. Aspirin did however do its appointed job very well in 39% of the trial subjects. It was the study's findings that "boosters" in the amount of aspirin taken would be necessary to adequately alleviate the problem of "platelet clumping." In the article published in the journal *Circulation* in February/98, Dr. Juana Valles and team, along with Dr. Aaron Marcus from *Cornell University Medical College* in New York, determined the following: to maintain inhibition, normal subjects required an intermittent (additional booster dose) of 500 mgs of aspirin every two weeks (aspirin stays in the system for 10-14 days); this regimen was supplemented with a regular, low maintenance dosage of 50 mgs ASA per day. The trial researchers wanted to avoid creating negative side effects by administering *too much daily maintenance* aspirin. The main side effects could be intestinal, stomach or possibly brain hemorrhage. Apparently, this regimen was successful in limiting the thrombotic effect by mediating the platelets binding or aggregating with red blood cells. It would seem that with added inherited, inflammatory or specific forms of *thrombopilia* and associated risk factors (particularly if they are undiscovered), it would become even more difficult to control platelet aggregation. There have also been other studies that indicated that low dose aspirin may not be sufficient in older patients with more advanced heart disease, and that for them higher doses may be required. I present this information for the patient's review and for discussion with their doctors. **Again, aspirin regimen, and particularly adding increased dosage, should <u>never be undertaken</u> without the doctor's agreement. This can be a slippery slope and requires monitoring by a physician. Just because it is sold over the counter doesn't mean there are not risks.**

## ASPIRIN AND RECURRENT STROKES

Doctor Vadim Karepov, M.D., Ph.D, from *Tel Aviv Medical Center* in Israel, working with his associates, studied 3,140 stroke patients. Of this total number, 901 had suffered a second stroke and 2,239 study subjects had experienced only the initial ischemic stroke. What they *discovered* from this trial was that aspirin had *failed* to accomplish the objective in 126 of the 2,239 patients who had experienced their first stroke. This overall number of 2,239 represents a significant enrollment. The researchers had given these test patients varying doses of aspirin, from daily amounts of 100 mgs to 1000 mgs. What the study ascertained was that patients with advanced lipid abnormalities, such as very high total cholesterol or very high individual lipid factors (as with LDL), stood a higher risk of aspirin failure than those with less severe hyperlipidemia. **These patients, according to the study, would benefit from higher doses of aspirin.** The findings were presented at the *American Heart Association's 21st International Joint Conference on Stroke and Cerebral Circulation.* Professor of Neurology Cathy Helgason M.D., from the *University of Illinois College of Medicine,* supporting the results of the Tel Aviv study, explained that additional studies on the effect of aspirin in preventing subsequent stroke recurrence in some patients while not in others, seem to corroborate the study findings. **Dr. Karepov** had stated, *"Our results show a possible way of preventing a second stroke in these patients who will require higher doses or other aggressive therapy."* The doctor went on to explain that aspirin's effectiveness increased with 350 mg/daily or even higher doses. The Israeli doctor also included the possible treatment with anticoagulants, even suggesting combination drug therapy. This idea came from Helgason's findings. "The study provides another piece of the puzzle as to why some people fail with aspirin." Helgason's conclusions further suggest that some are not taking the right doses, and that there might be a particular dose to be identified for each particular person. Drug therapy in such cases might include the drug Ticlid (a drug developed to reduce the sticking of platelets in patients prone to "platelet clumping"). Plavix is another of the newer favorite drugs. There are additional studies recommending low dose warfrin (Coumadin) in combination with aspirin. This particular study as well as those referenced would certainly raise the question as to whether someone with a high degree of atherosclerosis and general plaque presence should be administered as low a daily dosage of aspirin as 40 or 81 mgs.

# Chapter 49

# Arterial Spasms

We have all experienced harmless but annoying muscle twitches in the arm or leg or even in an eyelid. Similarly, a spasm can and often does occur in an artery itself at the arterial wall. Among patients with known or unknown fatty build-up within their arteries, the results of such an event can be very grave. This seemingly innocent flexing or spasmodic action within the artery can be compared to pinching one's fingers together with a sticky substance between them, creating a "crazy glue" effect; this serves as an elementary description of an "arterial spasm." Now, add the adhesive, negative qualities of "fibrin glue," or additional clotting factors, and one can develop a very "sticky" situation. All the more reason to learn your hidden risk factors, with careful attention to LDL cholesterol, fibrinogen and C-reactive protein. As we now understand, it is a combination of negative traits that often lead to final endpoints. Cigarette smokers have an increased risk for arterial spasms, and one Japanese study of coronary spasm found that 30% of those in the study who experienced arterial spasms had a mutation of a gene identified as the *eNOS* gene (endothelial nitric oxide synthase). The study was done at *Kumamoto University School of Medicine* in Kumamoto, Japan under the direction of Dr. Masafumi Nakayama. The researchers found that mutation of the gene reduces amounts of *nitric oxide,* which is the ultimate cause of the spasms (in this particular study). You might recall earlier reading that the amino acid L-arginine is a supplement accredited with the ability to increase the production of nitric oxide.

# Chapter 50

# Even NON-FAT DAIRY clogs Arteries

In August 1998 an article published by author WB Grant in *Alternative Medical Review* entitled **"Milk and other Dietary Influences on Coronary Heart Disease"** proved that milk (whether whole or nonfat) plays an active role in calcification of the coronary arteries. Adding to this information, a similar article in May 2000 in *Medical Hypotheses* by S. Seely proffered the theory that excessive milk intake would have a negative effect on circulation, as well as contributing to the coronary calcification process. Who would have thought that something as downright healthy as consuming non-fat milk could be harmful and involved in the actual calcification process? No doubt we will be hearing more about this area of investigation as time goes on. Apparently, milk is for babies!

## THE VALUE OF TREADMILL EXAMS

I recalled a fishing trip with two friends in central California in 1978. During our ride to the lake, one of the men mentioned that he was scheduled to have his annual physical. I suggested that after the physical, if the doctor said, "you should stand on the corner with a sign saying you are a picture of health" without suggesting a treadmill, (which was not then standard) you might do well to insist on one. In fact it happened almost exactly that way, and when my friend asked for the treadmill, the doctor said he didn't need one. "If you won't schedule me for one," my friend Mario explained, "I will have to go elsewhere to get it." The doctor ordered the treadmill and shut it down prematurely when the man couldn't continue past five minutes. He scheduled my friend for an angiogram, which discovered 2 significant blockages (one almost 90% and the other 50%), and a subsequent angioplasty procedure was performed. Question: If my friend had not become involved in his own healthcare, would he sooner or later have suffered a heart attack or even premature death? The other friend on that fishing trip did not have a stress test and, regrettably, passed away three years later from a diabetes-related heart attack. Whether or not the treadmill would have eliminated the second situation is now a non-issue.

## WHAT DID MICHAEL MILKIN LEARN ABOUT THE NEED FOR EARLY TESTING?

Michael Milkin, formerly known as the "junk bond king of Wall Street," went to his doctor requesting a PSA antigen test because a long-time friend had passed away thirty days before from prostate cancer. Milkin's doctor told the 46 year old man he was too young for a prostate test. Milkin insisted and got the test against the doctor's advice. The prognosis was that Milkin did indeed have prostate cancer, and he was given a prognosis of one year to eighteen months to live! New testing procedures and new information for that matter (as we have discussed earlier) have a long history of not being readily accepted into common practice. It is unfortunate for those patients caught in the nebulous interim time period. It almost seems like the profession and the insurance industry are saying, "Do we really need this?" Five or ten years later it would be unacceptable **not to administer** the same test whose application they previously rejected. We are really talking less about prostate cancer then we are prevention, but while we are on the subject there may be something here you might want to share with a friend dealing with prostate. An advancement known as *Proton Beam therapy* is in practice at *Loma Linda University Medical Center*, which is curing prostate cancer contained in the prostate almost miraculously, with only minor discomfort. The radiation dose is aimed strategically at the tumor where it focuses 76% of the total radiation on just the tumor itself, sparing surrounding tissue. It is also 46% more effective than traditional radiation. This equipment was built at a cost of $50 million and few patients are being told by their doctors of its availability, and many who would benefit from the procedure are not even aware of it. Milkin has since donated $25 million of his own money toward finding a cure for prostate cancer, and health-wise, he is reported to be doing very well after five years — only because a simple test alerted his physician.

# WITHOUT FINDING HIDDEN CAUSE, THE DESTRUCTION CONTINUES

Have you known someone who underwent bypass surgery and a few years (usually ten) down the line, the plumbing was again "stopping up?" Quite simply, without the source of the problem identified and mediated, the patient's health problems were destined to continue, eventually bringing the patient again to crisis even though it might take ten or fifteen years.

# Chapter 51

# Distinct Differences
## *between* FATS

Many people in an effort to "cut the fat" have to some degree been counterproductive in maximizing the benefit. There are three kinds of fat, and two of them are vital to our health. It is the saturated and trans fats that one wants to eliminate while honoring the beneficial attributes of the necessary *polyunsaturated and monounsaturated* fat types. Just as we as a public have had to learn to identify the three breakdowns in cholesterol, the LDL, HDL, and triglycerides, adding an understanding of the three distinctions of fats would be very beneficial, particularly for parents.

## THE GOOD FATS

- ▶ Polyunsaturated
- ▶ Monounsaturated

A study of particular interest to senior citizens;

Researchers in Italy found that
those trial subjects who consumed the most
monounsaturated fat, particularly the fat derived
from "extra virgin" olive oil, performed best on
mental exams testing cognitive function.

## BAD FATS

**TRANS FATS** are found in pastries, certain breads, fast foods, shortening, candies and among other prepared foods. The public at large has been told for years to prefer margarines over butter. This turned out to be a major case of misinformation. Stick margarine (the hard kind) rates much higher than actual butter in its harmful effects on the arteries. The process developed by manufacturer scientists almost a hundred years ago called *Hydrogenation* was welcomed with open arms by the food industry. The discovery of hydrogenation benefited the retailer because it would permit foodstuffs to remain on display shelves fresher and longer. It also enhanced the flavor of certain foods. It provided all these advantages and at the same time reduced the amount of spoilage. The wholesaler had fewer food products returned by the stores. It was, as you can imagine, a welcomed breakthrough. The problem is that the public and probably the food industry as a whole did not have a clue how much damage this process was doing to people's cardiovascular systems. Dr. Walter Willett, whose titles include Professor of Epidemiology and Nutrition, and Professor of Medicine at *Harvard Medical School and Harvard Public Health*, said last year that an estimated 30,000 people a year actually die prematurely as a result of *trans fat* intake. He added that epidemiological evidence suggests that the real number may be several times higher! Who might be the largest segment of the population ingesting this stuff? Our children. Germany apparently is one of two countries that have now banned trans fats from products on consumer shelves. Will the US soon follow suit, or will they be looking back 15 years from now admitting that we probably should have done something to protect our young people? This young group may be the most affected in our society because their diet is heavy in pizza, french fries, donuts, cookies, crackers, popcorn (flavored with hydrogenated butter) and other fast foods known to contain large amounts of trans fats. Unfortunately we adults have been irresponsible or unaware and a good deal responsible for feeding these products to our children. **As bad as saturated fats themselves are, their cousins, these *trans fats*, may be twice as dangerous.**

Even starkly reduced fat intake needs to be monitored. We still need a measure of fats, and strict vegetarians often experience an imbalance without knowing why. Fat from animal products (saturated fats) is what needs to be eliminated or minimized in the diet. The advice from the professionals is to definitely try to eliminate *trans fats* that are found in great amounts in coconut and palm oils. Be aware of them on labels and shun products with the killer phrase, **"partially hydrogenated,"** particularly if the words appear among the first few entrants listed. The ingredients most used in the product are supposed to be listed first.

## VERY BAD FATS

**SATURATED FATS** These fats also have been used extensively for many years in the manufacture of candies and pastries, often disguised under the names of *"hardened fats,"* or as ***partially hydrogenated*** oils. They are prevalent in meat and dairy products, poultry, cream, whole milk, cheese, eggs and butter. The type of fat is more important than the *total fat,* and saturated fats of animal origin are of course least desirable and most harmful.

Not only are the trans fats ugly, they are downright destructive, and what makes them even more offensive is that we as a society have not really been privy to their existence and the degree they can impact our cardiovascular health until fairly recently. To some degree the health community has been making the case, but people weren't listening. We have been told about the good guys, and are learning that the seemingly innocent process of converting soft or natural margarines and butters into convenient cubes, hydrogenating them into "hard butters and margarines," is anything but innocent. This word appearing on some labels triggers panic in the hearts of knowledgeable, health-conscious individuals who are concerned with what their children are being fed. Why have these *transfats* been served to an unsuspecting consumer? To begin with it should be noted that manufacturers have benefited significantly by the lower cost of using these destructive ingredients. There is also the real fact that *transfats* cause foods to remain fresher on grocery shelves, which pleases the manufacturer and the store chains and helps the bottom line. Governmental intervention to outlaw these ingredients in food processing (as was done in Germany) would be a valid goal.

# Chapter 52

# ALTERNATIVE
## *Medicine*

If you are an advocate of alternative medicine you are in a very elite group, according to a study that was published in the *Journal of American Medical Association* authored by John A. Astin, Ph.D, from *Stanford University*. The doctor concluded that people who subscribe to alternative medicine are better educated and have a more holistic approach to health than those patients who use only conventional medicine. Of the 1,000 participants in the study, 40% reported using some form of alternative health care during the preceding year. What is particularly interesting is that these people were not dissatisfied with or mistrustful of the doctors who attended them regularly. Apparently they see alternative medicine as an adjunct extension of their health care.

While traditional medicine has for years rejected medical claims coming from alternative medicine advocates, they have now been forced to acknowledge certain benefits and remedies. While their own alma maters have been graduating doctors with degrees in nutritional medicine, the "old school" has had, out of respect for their former universities (if for no other reason), been obligated to accept the knowledge that yes, vitamins and supplements are legitimate sources and adjunct therapy for modern medicine. Chiropractic, herbal supplements, and even massage techniques are being recommended when in the past they were not even considered legitimate therapy. Eastern medicine has been around more than 4,000 years and certainly even the strongest skeptic would have to assume that something beneficial was learned during all that time of experimentation. After all, the West is the youngster in this family of medical history. In certain Asian countries the standard of care is such that the doctor is only paid while the patient remains healthy and well. If the patient becomes ill, it follows that the doctor is not doing his job and not deserving of pay! Interesting concept? Not to be denied, the baby boomers spent an estimated $3.8 billion on herbs and other supplements in 1998. That number has only been growing to 2003. The Louis Harris survey reported that 96% of pharmacists found a very definite rise in demand for herbal supplements since 1994. This generation of baby boomers are not afraid to question, and not afraid to think on their own. According to John Cardellina, a chemist with the *Council for Responsible Nutrition*, "We are the generation that said, 'Never trust anyone over 30.'" According to Cardellina, "We don't want to get sick and we sure don't want to get old." I saw a hat on someone's head a couple of years ago that read, *"Old age sucks."* The good news is, now more than ever before much is out there to slow the process. Centurians are everywhere. Have you noticed how many young people you see today carrying water bottles? The evidence mounts daily that eight glasses of water, may absolutely be one of the most important things one can do to benefit one's health. Even doctors are taking supplements, herbs and more vitamins than ever before.

What is so strange is that the same profession that has denied, ignored and downright blasphemed alternative medicine is now, under the umbrella of their AMA organization, fighting to gain control of the billion-dollar vitamin industry, even asking Congress to amend the *Dietary Supplement Health and Education Act* to permit FDA oversight of the supplement and herbal remedy industries. There are also movements in progress to regulate vitamins by doctor prescription. Progress in another similar movement in Geneva, Switzerland was temporarily tabled in June of 1997 when Chancellor Kohl decided not (at least for the time being) to endorse the "Codex Cartel." According to Dr. Matthias Rath, Kohl was spearheading the *"Codex Alimentarius,"* an international pharmaceutical cartel, in an international effort to ban worldwide any health information relating to vitamins and other natural therapies. It is a fact that certain pharmaceutical companies are acquiring major positions or even buying vitamin companies outright to get in on the outstanding revenue bandwagon.

# Chapter 53

# Go Figure! A Drink Could Save Your Life!

When you hear of a study that includes as many as 21,537 test subjects, you can bet it is a pretty significant cross-section of people. So it was with a study called **"The largest study to look at alcohol consumption and cardiac death from light drinking."** The results from the *Harvard Medical School*, Boston, MA study were announced by the study's author, Dr. Christine Albert, and reported in a *Journal of the American Heart Association, Circulation.* One of the significant findings reported was that of the 21,537 healthy men who were followed for twelve years, 141 were lost to sudden death from cardiac arrest. The reporting doctor stated:

*" We found that the men who drank between 2 and 6 alcoholic beverages a week had a lower risk of sudden cardiac death compared to the men who never drank alcohol or those who drank 2 or more drinks a day. "*

Men who drank 2-4 or 6 drinks per week had a 60% and 79% lower risk of cardiac death respectively, compared with men who consumed two or fewer drinks per week.

These test subjects were healthy men who did not have pre-existing cardiovascular disease. The study author further reported that **cardiac risks rose as men began to drink *increasingly* more than these amounts.** "Our study found the risk **began to increase at more than two drinks per day,"** reported Dr. Albert. Obviously, this therapy is not recommended for those individuals with a drinking problem.

In January 2003, another *Harvard University Medical School* study led by Dr. Kenneth Mukamai found that *any* alcoholic beverage regardless of its source; beer, white/red wine, or liquor all offered some protection against heart attack. Remember, it was the contention a few years ago that red wine was the one beverage that would benefit patients. This was determined after studying the French consumption of red wine and fewer heart attacks. This new study found that **what** you drink is not as important as how **often** you drink it. Whether someone drank less than a half drink or whether they consumed four complete drinks a week the most benefit was found among those who drank frequently. The study confirmed a positive effect on sticky platelets. There are other ways to inhibit the sticking of platelets such as aspirin therapy. As an example it would be interesting to see a study comparing fish oil, aspirin, and alcohol's effect on platelets.

# Chapter 54

# A Physical
# FIT FOR A KING

If you were the president of the United States or an actual king you would be assured of having the most complete thorough physical examination possible. All the stops would be pulled out and expense would not be an issue. Our presidents receive their annual physicals at the *Bethesda Naval Station* in Maryland. If you were a president or a *real king*, your physical would include the latest technology and diagnostic testing available. As a matter of fact, our sitting President was given a full body scan during his last physical. You *are* the king or queen in your domain and among your family—do you or your loved ones deserve any less of a quality physical than the one reserved for a real king? Let's review what is involved in an average physical.

# THE POOR MAN'S PHYSICAL

You will be asked upon your arrival to take a seat in the waiting room and fill out the forms the staff member gives you. We all know the drill. The questions about your family history, if you have had surgeries, medications you might currently be on, and if you have had adverse reaction to any antibiotics. You will be given an EKG to determine if you have had a previous silent heart attack or if in fact you are exhibiting electrical heart rhythm irregularities. Your temperature, weight and blood pressure will also be documented. Now your big moment has arrived as you prepare to meet OZ! You might pop a breath mint in anticipation of the opportunity you will no doubt be given to open your mouth and roar ahhhh! As new patients, we always want to make a real good first impression. Now somewhere about now, you look up to see the doctor coming across the room wielding that formidable irritating tomahawk which doctors promptly whack you with several times to duly challenge your reflexes. You probably wonder if this is really necessary as it seems to be an important ritualistic part of each annual physical. Now your body will be non-invasively probed in certain areas and attention paid to the size of internal organs and tenderness or soreness as well. Your lungs will be listened to from the front and rear. The doctor will listen to your heart for murmurs, heart beat and rhythm disturbances. If he or she is conscientious, they will listen to your carotid arteries to ascertain if there is appreciable stenosis. The long awaited words inform you it is time to get dressed. The nurse will send you to the lab to have some blood drawn and you will dutifully pee in the bottle. The blood work will include the standard CBC overall panel. Dr. Oz will thank you for coming in, explaining that you will receive a call when the results of the blood work become available. You may not have been evaluated for C-reactive protein (although in 2003 you might), nor will you be tested for fibrinogen, LP (a) apolipoprotein ratios, low grade infections, coronary calcification, homocysteine or many of the other risk factors for heart disease and stroke that we have been discussing. Cholesterol may or may not have been assayed. You have had half a physical in keeping with the insurance guidelines and restrictions.

## THE KING'S PHYSICAL

Here, price will not be an issue, nothing is going to be spared. Nothing because, after all, no doctor would want to lose a king or a world leader on their watch. Speaking of kings, while Enrico Caruso, the world's undisputed King of Grand Opera was lying on his death bed in Rome, the doctors refused to operate on him for fear they might be unsuccessful and lose Italy's and the world's favorite singer. According to the singer's wife Dorothy Caruso, as she later wrote in her memoirs, the attending doctors did not want to try anything desperate to save her husband fearing they might still lose their famous client and their reputations would hang in the balance. To lose such an illustrious patient would not only be bad for one's career, but no doubt very unhealthy for the patient as well. So let us observe what the preventive leading-edge physician of the 21st century might concern themselves with in the evaluation of their kingly patients and hopefully you and your family.

# APPOINTMENT WITH DR. FEELGOOD

This modern doctor's presentation might begin some-thing like this. *"Like any physician I get very upset if I lose a patient to any disease but particularly to heart disease because there is so much new information to prevent it. I realize that to some of my colleagues and insurance providers, I am considered a little extreme in my preventive care of my patients.* I have just read your family history from the form you have prepared for me to learn if there has been any heart disease or stroke related illness among your immediate family, siblings, par-ents, uncles, aunts, grandparents. Where my examination differs from the typical physical you have had in the past is that I don't give a damn about what your HMO ap-proves. If I think it is something necessary that would benefit you, I am going to order it. Certain tests that are available now may not be added to the insurance com-pany recommended list for another ten years. I want what is best for you and your family today. If we find after examining you for any of the inherited risk factors that you are positive for one or more, I am going to suggest that we run similar tests on your children. To some of my colleagues this may also sound a little extreme but many of the mechanisms of heart disease are acknowledged to be of an inherited nature. These risk factors very often run in a family and begin very early in life. The same mecha-nisms we might have identified in a parent's profile could be the same risks inherent in their offspring. Wouldn't it make sense to intervene on their behalf and spare them the ravages of heart disease later in life? This approach is called *Preventive Cardiology*. The other kind that deals with the advanced disease may be called *Interventional Cardiology*. The blood tests I will be ordering for you are a complete battery to cover the latest risk factors. I see you have not had a *colonoscopy* and you are over 50, let's schedule one for you. I don't believe in just doing a *sigmoidoscopy* to save the money waiting until you become symptomatic.

If you are wondering how I know that this preventive approach is the correct one, let me answer your concern with a question. Even if it were wrong to suggest testing you for the hidden traits, or to ask you to take a natural vitamin or supplement to neutralize one or more of the traits, what harm would these things do? My creed is to do no harm. My worry is over how much harm I will actually permit if I ignore what in my heart and mind I believe should be done right now. Yes, I believe there are benefits in full body scans.

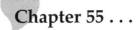Chapter 55 . . .

# *Removing* Heart Disease
## *from its*
# #1 POSITION

It is with serious contemplation, and after five years of research, that I make the following observation. I believe there is a concept that many knowledgeable leaders in the field of cardiology are for the first time beginning to consider, but are not yet prepared to verbalize publicly. A professional hesitates, necessarily, to put his or her reputation with colleagues at risk by engaging in speculation. These are men and women of science, and daring to dream is not of itself a scientific principle. You and I, however, have that luxury. I believe it can now be legitimately argued on the evidence that **if the advice of the leaders** whose work you have been presented with were implemented at the earliest time in our youngsters lives, and preventive blood tests and appropriate controls put in place along with proper diet and exercise, non-congenital heart disease could be reduced to manageable proportions within one or two generations. The reduced cost to healthcare as a result of a preventive approach would be staggering, as this killer would be denied its current number one position. Most importantly, the number of lives saved from premature death would be almost overwhelming to envision and therefore, too far a departure from current thinking to be embraced and accepted at this time.

---

*One of the greatest pains to human nature is the pain of a new idea. It...makes one think that after all, your favorite notions may be wrong, your firmest beliefs ill-founded.* —**Walter Bagehot 1864**

# GLOSSARY

**AAA,** abdominal aortic aneurysm

**ACE inhibitors,** an angiotensin blood pressure medication

**Aerosols,** tiny droplets of bodily fluid expelled in a sneeze or cough

**ALT—(SGPT),** a measurement of liver enzyme

**Alzheimers,** a disease robbing the elderly of mental function

**Anaphylactic shock,** causing life threatening drops in blood pressure

**Aneurysm,** a bulge within a heart or brain artery

**Angina,** "heart pain" from blood starvation

**Angiogenesis,** the body's natural bypass of growing tiny vessels around blockages

**Angiograms,** utilize a tiny camera to view the inside of arteries

**Angioplasty,** a procedure that opens an obstructed artery by balloon inflation

**Antibodies,** marker of prior infection

**Antioxidants,** fight oxidation and enhance immune system.

**Aortic valve sclerosis,** thickening, scarring, stiffening of the valve leaflets

**Aortic valve stenosis,** diseased and narrowed aortic valve

**Aortic valve,** main heart valve located in the aorta

**Arrhythmia,** irregular heartbeat

**Arterioles,** tiny vessels that grow to permit blood around a blockage

**Arteriosclerosis,** hardening of the arterial walls

**AST, (SGOT),** liver enzymes increased with liver damage and inflammation

**Asymptomatic,** not showing symptoms

**Atheroma,** fatty degeneration of the inner arterial wall

**Atherosclerosis,** cholesterol and fatty deposit buildup in the coronary arteries

**Atrial fibrillation,** atrium beating out of control and rhythm with the rest of the heart

**Atrium,** upper heart chamber receiving blood from the veins sending it to the ventricles

**Basophils,** battle against allergies

**Beta-carotene,** antioxidant containing vitamin a

**Brain attack,** a mini (TIA), or major stroke

**By-pass,** a surgery replacing diseased coronary arteries with leg arteries

**Calcification,** deposits of calcium into tissues

**Cardiologists,** medical doctors specializing in care of the cardio-vascular system

**Cardiomyopathy,** chronic damaged heart muscle from disease or enlargement

**Cardio-thoracic surgeon,** a surgeon who operates on the heart and lungs

**Carotid arteries,** the arteries in the neck leading to the brain

**CBC,** (Complete Blood Count), blood chemistry panel

**Chlamydia pneumoniae,** a bacterial disease caused by upper respiratory illness

**CMV,** (cytomegalovirus), of the herpes family

**Coenzyme Q 10,** required by every cell in the body

**Cognitive function,** elements of mental function

**Collateral vessels,** another name for "natural bypass"

**C-reactive protein,** a marker of bodily inflammation

**CRP,** C-reactive protein

**Dementia,** loss of brain function, shrinking of the brain

**Diabetes Mellitus,** a vascular disorder of carbohydrate metabo-lism, a vascular disease

**Diagnostic,** test to determine illness or wellness

**Diuretics,** promote urination of fluid and salts

**Doppler ultrasound,** a technology using sound waves to measure obstruction

**Drug resistant,** a disease that has built an immunity to available medication

**DVT,** deep vein thrombosis, clots formed within the legs and recesses of the calf

**Dysfunction,** not functioning as normal

**Dyslipidemia,** out of control cholesterol levels

**EBCT,** Electronic beam computed tomography

**Echocardiogram,** uses sound waves to observe shapes and certain organ functions

**Edema,** accumulation of fluid in blood vessels in legs and abdomen

**Ejection fraction,** the measurement of how the blood is forced from the heart to the body

**EKG,** electrocardiogram, a machine that records the electrical function of the heart

**Electrophoresis,** study of HDL and LDL components

**Embolic,** as related to an embolism

**Embolism,** a sudden obstruction of clot formation

**Embolus,** a particle that circulates in the blood

**Endarterectomy,** serious surgery to open carotid blockage

**Endocarditis,** an infection of the heart valves or lining

**Endothelium,** fine smooth linings of the arteries

**Epidemiology,** identifies and controls disease outbreak

**Fetal neural,** spinal malformation of a baby's spine

**Fibrates,** a form of cholesterol drug most effective for triglyceride and HDL dysfunction

**Fibrillation,** beating out of sync and rhythm

**Fibrin,** formed from fibrinogen in clot formation

**Fibrinogen,** a blood protein involved in stroke and plaque produced by the liver converted to fibrin with calcium present

**Fibrinolysis,** process of enzymatic breakdown of fibrin

**Fictional,** imagined but not true

**Folic acid,** of the B complex family, folate

**Framingham Study,** early government heart study

**H. pylori,** a bacterial infection suspect in heart disease

**Hardening of the arteries,** arteriosclerosis

**HCM,** (hypertrophic cardiomyopathy),

**HDL,** high density lipoprotein (good cholesterol)

**HeFH,** hypercholesterolemia, a rare childhood disease

**Hemorrhagic,** prone to excessive bleeding

**Hidden risks,** not normally found during routine exams

**HMO,** health managed organization

**Homocysteine,** a sulphur containing byproduct of methionine

**Homocysteininemia,** high (hcy) possibly heredity related

**Hypertension,** high blood pressure

**Hypertrophic cardiomyopathy,** thickening of heart walls

**Inflammatory markers,** tests that record inflammation

**Inherited,** a risk factor of genetic origin

**Insulin,** a hormone produced by the pancreas involved with diabetes

**Ischemia,** a reduction in normal flow of the blood to the heart

**IVUS,** intravascular ultrasound

**JAMA,** Journal of the American Heart Association

**L-arginine,** an amino acid

**L-carnitine,** an amino acid

**l-cysteine,** an amino acid

**LDL,** low density lipoprotein (bad)

**Leukocytes,** white blood cells

**Lipoprotein (a),** a negative component of the LDL structure

**L-lysine,** an amino acid

**LP little a**, a detrimental component of the LDL cholesterol structure

**Lumen,** the open area within an artery

**Lutein,** from green leafy vegetables helpful for eyes and arteries

**Macula degeneration,** leading cause of blindness among seniors

**Metabolic process,** affected by metabolism

**Methionine,** a sulfur containing amino acid

**Mevacor,** (lovastatin) the first statin drug

**Minimally invasive,** opening only the smallest area necessary during surgery

**Mitral valve,** one of four heart valves

**Monocytes,** process damaged or dead cells

**Monounsaturated fats,** a good fat

**MRSA,** *(methicillin-resistant staph aureus)* found in hospitals, **retirement homes**

**Multi-vessel heart disease,** occurring within more than one artery

**Mycoplasma,** pneumonia

**Myocarditis,** a bacterial infection affecting heart muscle through inflammation

**N-acetylcysteine,** an amino acid

**Natural by-pass,** body's ability to grow smaller vessels around a blockage

**Neutrophils,** primary agents against infection

**Niacin,** vitamin B3, also known as nicotinic acid and the trade name niaspan

**Niaspan,** a prescribed form of time release niacin

**Nicotinic acid,** Vitamin B3

**NO,** (nitric oxide) made from nitrogen gas

**Non-invasive,** procedures that do not enter the body

**Novel,** uncommon

**Nuclear treadmill,** utilizes a liquid agent to trace blood flow to all areas of the heart

**Occlusion,** blockage in an artery

**Omega 3,** an important oil beneficial against heart attack and stroke

**PAD,** (peripheral artery disease)

**Pathologist,** whose science deals with tissues

**Peripheral artery disease,** (PAD) heart disease extended beyond the coronary arteries

**Pernicious anemia,** a rare but serious form of anemia

**Plaque,** the buildup of fat deposits within the arteries or vessels

**Platelet aggregation,** sticking of platelets together

**Polyunsaturated fat,** a good fat

**Postmortem,** after death

**Predisposition,** prone to as in family inherited traits

**Prenisone,** a popular steroid

**Prognosis,** what is medically expected

**Prophylaxis,** a preventive

**Pulmonary embolism,** a blood clot in the lung or lung artery

**Regimen,** a planned therapy

**Regurgitating blood**, blood flow rejected by a diseased heart valve

**Remethylation,** reconstituted

**Re-stenosis,** a repeated obstruction or blockage

**Saturated,** undesirable fats from animal sources

**Silent heart attack,** occurring without symptoms or without knowledge

**Silent ischemia,** diminished blood flow not obvious symptomatically to the patient

**Silent stroke,** one occurring to areas of the brain that do not show symptoms

**Sleep apnea,** a sleep condition where the breathing stops due to obstructed airway

**Staph infection,** *staphylococcus aureus* contracted through an open incision

**Stenosis,** obstruction or blockage

**Stents,** small metal sleeves inserted into an artery to keep it open

**Subfractions,** more specific and accurate breakdown of LDL and HDL cholesterol

**Superbugs,** drug resistant germs or bacteria

**Syndrome X,** an endangering combination of factors in diabetes

**Synthesis,** process of creating a substance from a combination of materials

**Thallium treadmill,** utilizes a tracing agent to follow blood flow throughout the heart

**Thrombosis,** resulting from development and collection of a clot within an artery

**Thrombus,** a stationary clot clinging to its point of origin

**Thromophilia,** multiple factors affecting blood clotting and flow

**TIA,** (temporary ischemic attack), a mini stroke, precursor of major stroke

**TMG,** (tri-methyl glycine)

**Trans fats,** dangerous form of processed fat

**Triglycerides,** made from stored sugars and fats circulating in the blood

**Ultra-fast CT,** a CT scan that captures pictures between heart beats

**Unstable plaque,** usually soft in composition and ready to dislodge at anytime

**Vascular diseases,** affecting the heart arteries and vascular system

**Ventricle fibrillation,** the ventricle flutters out of time

**Ventricle,** receives blood from the upper atrium, sends it to the arteries

**Viscosity,** thickness of the blood

**Vulnerable plaque,** plaque very prone to dislodge and rupture

**WBC,** (White Cell Count)

**Widow maker,** left main ventricle where most major heart attacks strike

ADDITIONAL REFERENCES TO THOSE APPEARING IN TEXT

## C-REACTIVE PROTEIN, (CRP)
*Koenig W.*
Comparison of C-reactive protein and low-density lipoprotein cholesterol levels in the prediction of first cardiovascular events. N Engl J Med. 2002 Nov 14;347(O20):1557-65.
*Jialal I, Devaraj S.*
C-reactive protein and myocardial infarction. J Clin Epidemiol. 2002 May;55(5):445-5
*Farmer JA, Torre-Amione G.*
Inflammation and atherosclerosis: the value of the high-sensitivity C-reactive protein assay as a risk marker. Am J Clin Pathol. 2001 Dec;116 Suppl:S108-15. Review227.
*Wong BY, Gnarpe J, Teo KK, Ohman EM, Prosser C, Gibler WB, Langer A, Chang WC, Armstrong PW.*
Atherosclerosis and inflammation. Curr Atheroscler Rep. 2002 Mar;4(2):92-8.
*Vecsei PV, Kircher K, Reitner A, Khanakah G, Stanek G.*
*Ridker, P.M., Buring, J.E. cook, N.r. Rifai, N. (2003. C-reactive Protein, the Metabolic Syndrome, and risk of Incident Cardiovascular Events: An 8-year Follow-up of 14719 Initially Healthy Women, Circuation 107: 391-397*
*Ridker, P.M., (2003. Clinical Application of C Reactive Protein for Cardiovascular Disease Detection and Prevention. Circulation 107: 363-369.*
*Yeung, A.C. Tsao, P. (2002). Statin Therapy: Beyond Cholesterol Lowering and Antiinflammatory Effects. Circulation 105: 2937-2938*
*Plenge, J. K., Hernandez, T.L., Weil, K.M., P.M Poirer, P., Grunwald, G.K., Marcovina, S.M., Eckel R.H. (2002). Simvastatin Lowers C-Reactive Protein Within 14 Days: An Effect Independent of Low-Density Lipoprotein Cholesterol Reduction. Circulation 106: 1447-1452.*
*D.A.M., Nijhuis, R.L.G., Hofman, A. Witteman, J.C.M.(2002). LongTerm Effects of Atherosclerosis Measured at Various Sites in the Arterial Tree: The Rotterdam Study. Stroke 33: 2750-2755 Ridker, P.M.*

## FIBRINOGEN
Association of plasma Fibrinogen levels with coronary artery disease, smoking and inflammatory markers deMaat MP, Pietersma A. Kofflard M, Siuiter W, Kluft C
*Voster HH, Venter CS.*
Why fibriogen should be measured as part of the coronary heart disease risk profile.
S Afr Med J. 1993 May;83(5):309-10. No abstract available.
*Smith FB, Lowe GD, Lee AJ, Rumley A, Leng GC, Fowkes FG*
Smoking, hemorheologic factors, and progression of peripheral arterial disease in patients with claudication.
J Vasc Surg. 1998 Jul:28(1):129-35.
*Meade TW.*
Fibrinogen and cardiovascular disease.
J Clin Pathol. 1997 Jan;50(1):13-5
*Ernst E.*
Fibrinogen
BMJ. 1991 Sep 14;303(6803):596-7
*Lee AJ, Fowkes FG, Rattray A, Rumley A, Lowe GD.*
Haemostatic and rheological factors in intermittent claudication: the influence of smoking and extent of arterial disease.
Br J Haematol. 1996 Jan;92(1):226-30
*Benzaquen LR, Yu H, Rifai N.*
Von Wilebrand factor and coronary heart disease. Prospective study and meta-analysis.
Eur Heart J. 2002 Nov 15;23(22):1764-70.

DeMaat MP, Kastelein JJ, Jukema JW, Zwinderman AH, Jansen H, Groenemeier B, Bruschke AV, Kluft C.
-455G/A polymorphism of the beta-fibrinogen gene is associated with the progression of coronary atherosclerosis in sysmptomatic men: proposed role for an acute-phase reaction pattern of fibrinogen. REGRESS group. Arterioscler Thromb Vasc Biol 1998 Feb;18(2):265-71.

Smith FB, Lee AJ, Hae CM, Rumley A, Lowe GD, Fowkes FG.
Plasma fibrinogen, haemostatic factors and prediction of peripheral arterial disease in the Edinburgh Artery Study.
Blood Coagul Fibrinolysis 2000 Jan;11(1):43-50.

Fowkes FG.
Fibriogen and peripheral arterial disease.
Eur Heart J. 1995 Mar;16 Suppl A:36-40; discussion 40-1. Review.
PNID: 7796829

Lowe G, Rumley A.
Clinical benefit of fibrinogen evaluation.
Blood Coagul Fibrinolysis. 1999 Feb;10 Suppl 1:S87-9.

Resch KL, Ernst E.
Fibrinogen and viscosity; risk factors for cardiovascular events.
Compr Ther. 1994;20(3):170-3.

Humphries SE, Luong LA, Ogg MS, Hawe E, Miller GJ.
The interleukin-6 −174 G/C promoter polymorphism is associated with risk of coronary heart disease and systolic blood pressure in healthy men. Eur Heart J 2001;22(24):2243-

Bielak LF, Klee GG, Sheedy PF, et al.
Association of fibrinogen with quantity of coronary artery calcification measured by electron beam computed tomography, Arterioscler Thromb Vase Biol (United States), Sep 2000,29(9):p2167-71

Benderly M, Graff E, Reicher-Reiss H, et al.
Fibrinogen is a predictor of mortality in coronary heart disease patients. The Bezafibrae Infarction Prevention (BIP) Study Group.

Lind P, Hedblad B, Stavenow L, et al.
Influence of plasma fibrinogen levels on the incidence of myocardial infarction and death is modified by other inflammation-sensitive proteins: a long-term cohort study.
Arterioscler Thromb Vasc Biol (United States), Mar 2001,21(3).

Salomaa V, Rasi V, Kulathinal S, et al.
Eriksson M, Egberg N, Warmala S, et al.
Relationship between plasma fibrinogen and coronary heart disease in women.
Arterioscler Thromb Basc Biol (United States),k Jan 1999, 19(1)p67-72.

Levenson J, Giral P, Megnien JL, et al.
Fibrinogen and its relations to subclinical extracoronary and coronary atherosclerosis in hypercholesterolemic men.
Arterioscler Thromb Vasc Biol (United States), Jan 1997, 17(1)P45-50.

Oosthuizen W, et al.
Both fish oil and olive oil lowered plasma fibrinogen in women with high baseline fibrinogen levels. Thromb Haemost 1994 Oct;72(4):557-62.
 Radcliffe Infirmary. Eur Heart J, 16 Suppl A(-HD-):42-5;discussion 45-6 1995 Mar.

Fowkes FG.
Recent progress in the clinical aspects of fibrinogen. Eur Heart J. 1995 Mar;16 Suppl A:54-91296.

Torgano G, Cosentini R,k Mandelli C, Perondi R, Blasi F, Bertinieri G, Tien TV, Ceriani G, Tarsia P, Arosio C, Ranzi ML.
Socioeconomic conditions in childhood and ischaemic heart disease during middle age. BMJ. 1990 Nov 17;301(6761):1121-3.

Sweetman PM, Thomas HF, Yarnell JW, Beswick AD, Baker IA, Elwood PC.
Lowering fibrinogen levels: clinical updae. BIP Study Group. Benzafibrate Infarction
Prevention. Blood Coagul Fibrinolysis. 1999 Feb;10 Suppl 1:S41-3.

Kaftan AH KaftanO.
Social determinants of von willebrand factor: the Whitehall II study. Arterioscler Thromb
Vasc Biol. 2000 Jul;20(7):1842-7.

Ferrie JE, Shipley MJ, Davey Smith G, Stansfeld SA, Marmot MG.
Fibrinogen, Viscosity and the 10-year incidence of ischaemic heart disease. Eur Heart J. 1996
Dec;17(12):1814-20.

Sansfeld SA, Fuhrer R, Shipley MJ, Marmot MG.
Change in health inequalities among British civil servants: the Whitehall II study. J
Epidemiol Community Health. 2002 Dec;56(12):922-6.

Ageno W, Finazzi S, Steidl L, Biotti MG, Mera V, Melzi D'Eril G, Venco A.
Psychological distress as a risk factor for coronary heart disease in the Whitehall II Study.
Int J Epidemiol. 2002. Feb;31(1):248-55.

Mattila K, Vasanen M, Valtonen V, Nieminen M, Palosuo T, Rasi V, Asikainen S.
Fibrinogen and risk of cardiovascular disease. The Framingham Study. JAMA. 1987 Sep
4;258(9):1183-6.

Van der Bom JG, de Maat MP, Bots ML, Haverkate F, de Jong PT, Hofman A, Kluft C,
Interindividual and intraindividual variability in plasma fibrinogen, TPA antigen, PAI
activity, and CRP in healthy, young volunteers and patients with angina pectoris.
Arterioscler Thromb Basc Biol (United States), Sep 1996, 16(9)p1156-62

Zito F, Di Castelnuovo A, Amore C, et al.
Bcl l polymorphism in the fibrinogen beta-chain gene is associated with the risk of familial
myocardial infarction by increasing plasma fibrinogen levels. A case-control study in a
sample of GISSI=2 patients.
Arterioscler Thromb Vasc Biol (United States), Dec 1997, 17(12)p3489-94.

Bielak LF, Klee GG, Sheedy PF, et al.
Association of fibrinogen with quantity of coronary artery calcification measured by elec-
tron beam computed tomography.
Arterioscler Thromb Vasc Biol (United States), Sep 2000, 20(9)p2167-71.

Folsom AR, Wu KK, Rasmussen M, et al.
Determinants of population changes in fibrinogen and factor VII over 6 years; the Athero-
sclerosis Risk in Communities (ARIC) Study.
Arterioscler Thromb Vasc Biol (United States), Feb 2000, 20(2)p601-6.

Benderly M, Graff E, Reicher-Reiss H, et al.
Fibrinogen is a predictor of mortality in coronary heart disease patients. The Bezafibrante
Infarction Prevention (BIP) Study Group
Arterioscler Thromb Vasc Biol (United States), Mar 1996, 16(3) p351

## CHLAMYDIA PNEUMONIAE

Coronary artery disease and infection with chlamydia pneumoniae. Jpn Heart J. 2000
Mar;41(2):165-72.472.

Ridker PM, Rifai N, Rose L, Buring JE, Cook NR.
Inflammatory bio-markers and cardiovascular risk prediction. J Intern Med. 2002
Oct;252(4):283-94.

Does chronic Chlamydia pneumoniae infection increase the risk of myocardial injury?
Insights from patients with non-ST-elevation acute coronary syndromes. Am Heart J. 2002
Dec;144(6):987-94.

Parager M, Turel Z, Speidl WS, Zorn G, Kaun C, Niessner A, Heinze G, Huk I, Maurer G,
Huber K, Wojta J.
Chlamydia pneumoniae and atherosclerosis. Actas Chir Belg. 2002 Oct;102(5):317-22.

_Leowattana W, Bhuripanyo K. Singhaviranon L, Akaniroj S., Mahanonda N, Samranthin M, Pokum S._
Chlamydia pneumoniae as an emerging risk factor in cardiovascular disease. JAMA. 2002 Dec4;288(21):2724-31. Review 206.
_Burczynski F, Hasinoff B, Zhong G._
Roxithromycin in prevention of acute coronary syndrome associated with chlamydia pneumoniae infection: a randomized placebo controlled trial. J Med Assoc Thai. 2001 Dec;84 Suppl 3:S669-75G.
_Kalayoglu MV, Libby P, Byrne GI._
Infection of monocytes with chlamydia(e). Microbiology. 2002 Dec;148(Pt 12):3955-9.
_Eowattana W._
The association of seropositivity to Helicobacter pylori, Chlamydia pneumoniae, and cytomegalovirus with risk of cardiovascular disease: a prospective study. J Am Coll Cardiol. 2002 Oct 16:40(8):1408-13.
_Maisch B, schonian U, Crombach M, Wendl I, Bethge C, Herzum M, Klein HH._
Chronic infections and atherosclerosis. J Med Assoc Thai. 2001 Dec;84 Suppl 3:S650-7.203.
_Fong IW, Chiu B, Vira E, et al._
Rabbit model for Chlamydia pneumoniae infection. J Clin Microbiol 1997, 35:48-52.
_Muhlstein JB, Anderson JL, Hammond EH et al._
Infection with Chlamydia pneumoniae accelerates the development of atherosclerosis and treatment with azithromycin prevents it in a rabbit model. Circulation 1998, 97:633-636.
_Gaydos, CA, Summersgill JT, Sahney NN, et al._
Replication of Chlamydia pneumoniae in vitro in human macrophages, endothelial cells and aortic artery smooth muscle cells. Infect Immun 1996, 64:1614-1620.
_Cunningham AF, Johnston SL, Julious SA, et al._
Chronic Chalmydia pneumoniae infection and asthma exacerbations in children. Eur Resp J 1998, 11:345-349.
_Wong, YK, Sueur JM, Fall CHD et al._
The species specificity of the microimmunofluorescence antibody test and comparisons with a time resolved fluoroscopic immunoassay for measuring IgG antibodies against Chlamydia pneumoniae J Clin Pathol 1999, 52:99-102.
_Kuo CC, Shor A, Campbell LA et al._
Demonstration of Chlamydia penumoniae in atherosclerotic lesions of coronary arteries. J Infect Dis 1993, 167:841-849.
_Campbell LA, O'Brien ER, Cappuccio AL, et al._
Detection of Chlamydia pneumoniae TWAR in human coronary atherectomy tissues. J Infect Dis 1995, 172:585-588
_Davidson M, Kuo CC, Middaugh JP, et al._
Confirmed previous infection with Chlamydia pneumoniae (TWAR) and its presence in early coronary atherosclerosis. Circulation 1998, 98:628-633. [Medline]
_Patel P, Mendall MA, Carrington D, et al._
Association of Helicobacter pylori and Chlamydia pneumoniae infections with coronary heart disease and cardiovascular risk factors. Brit Med J 1995, 311:711-714.
_Anderson JL, Cariquist JF, Muhlestine JB, et al._
Evaluation of C-reactive protein, an inflammatory marker and infectious serology as risk factors for coronary artery disease.
_John Ijem, JD; Carrie Granlie, PharmD_
More Than Cholesterol: The Complexity of Coronary Artery Disease
South Dakota Journal of Medicine, Volume 53, number 11; November 2000, p489
_Cushman M, Lemaitre RN, Kuller LH, Psaty BM, Macy EM, Sharrett AR, Tracy RP._
Treatment of Helicobacter pylori and Chlamydia pneumoniae infections decreases fibrinogen plasma level in patients with ischemic heart disease. Circulation. 1999 Mar 30;99(12):1555-9.

Kaftan AH, Kaftan O.
Coronary artery disease and infection with chalmydia pneumonia. Jpn Heart J. 2000 Mar;41(2):165-72.
Kaftan AH, Kahtan O.
Coronary artery disease and infection with chlamydia pneumonia. Jpn Heart J. 2000 Mar;41(2):165-72.
Muhlestein Joseph B, MD.
University of Utah School of Medicine, LDS Hospital
The Link Between Chlamydia pneumoniae and Atherosclerosis. Infect Med 14(5):380-382,392,426, 1997. \ \
Studies Link Chlamydia and Asthma. Pediatric News 31(4):17, 1998 1998 International. Chlamydia pneumoniae Infection and Atherosclerotic Coronary Disease.

## NITRIC OXIDE
Am J Physiol Heart Circ Physiol 2000 Dec;279(7):H2649-57f
Simvastatin upregulates coronary vascular endothelial nitric oxide production in conscious dogs.Falk E,
Shah PK, Fuster V..
Coronary plaque disruption. Circulation, 1995;92-657-671.
Castelli W.
Lipids risk factors, and ischemic heart disease. Atherosclerosis, 1996;124-S1-S9.
Heath KE, Humphries SE, Middleton-PriceH, Boxer M.
A molecular genetic service for diagnosing individuals with familial hypercholesterolaemia (FH) Eur J Hum Gen 2001;9:244-252
Jeziorska M, McCollum C, Woolley DE.
Mast cell distribution, activation, and phenotype in atherosclerotic lesions of human carotid arteries. J Pathol. 1997;183-248], j Pathol, 1997;182:115-122.

## CORONARY CALICIFICATION
Stephen Achenbach, MD et al.
Influence of Lipid-Lowering Therapy on the Progression of Coronary Artery Calcification
Lewis Wexler, MD, Chair; Bruce Brundage, MD; John Crouse, MD; Robert Detrano, MD, PhD; Valentin Fuster, MD, PhD; Jamshid Maddahi, MD; John Rumberger, MD, PhD; William Stanford, MD; Richard White, MD, Members; Kathryn Taubert, PhD, AHA Staff
Coronary Artery Calcification: Pathophysiology, Epidemiology, Imaging Methods, and Clinical Implications.
Rumberger JA, Simons DB, Fitzpatrick LA, et al.
Coronary artery calcium area by electron-beam computed tomography and coronary athero-sclerotic plaque area; a histopathologic correlative study. Circulation, 1995;92:2157-2162.
Agatston AS, Janowitz WR, Hildner FJ, et al.
Quantification of coronary artery calcium using ultrafast computed tomography. J Am Coll Cardiol, 1990;15:827-832.
Maher JE, Bielak LF, Raz JA, et al.
Progression of coronary artery calcification: a pilot study, Mayo Clin Proc. 1999;74:337
Callister TQ, Raggi P, Cooil B, et al.
Effect of HMG-CoA reductase inhibitors on coronary artery disease as assessed by electron-beam computed tomography. N Engl J Med. 1998;339:1972-1978.
Warren R. Janowitz, MD, Arthur S. Agatston, MD, Glenn Kaplan, Manuel Viamonte, Jr., Differences in Prevalence and Extent of Coronary Artery Calcium Detected by Ultrafast Computed Tomography in Asymptomatic Men and Women. Am J Cardiol 1993;72:247
Rumberger JA, Simons DB, Fitzpatrick LA, et al.
Coronary artery calcium area by electron-beam computed tomography and coronary athero-sclerotic plaque area; a histopathologic correlative study. Circulation, 1995;92:2157-2162.

Sangiorgi G, Rumberger JA, Severson A, et al.
Arterial calcification and not lumen stenosis is highly correlated with atherosclerotic plaque burden in humans: a histologic study of 723 coronary artery segments using nondecalcifying methodology. J Am Coll Cardiol. 1998;31:126-133.

Callister TQ, Raggi P, Cooil B, et al.
Effect of HMG-CoA reductase inhibitors on coronary artery disease as assessed by electron-beam commuted tomography N Engl I Med 1998:339: 1972-1978.

Budoff MJ, Lane KL, Bakhsheshi H, et al.
Rates of progression of coronary calciuim by electron beam tomography. Am J Cardiol, 2000;86:8-11.

Fitzpatrick LA, Severson A, Edweards WD, et al.
Diffuse calcification in human coronary arteries, association of osteopontin with atherosclerosis. J Clin Invest. 1994;94:1597-1604.

Doherty TM, Detrano RC.
Coronary arterial calcificaiton as an active process: a new perspective on an old problem. Calcif Tissue Int. 1994; 54:224-230.

Bvostrom K, Demer LL.
Regulatory mechanisms in vascular calcificaiton. Crit Rev Eukaryot Gene Expr. 2000;12:151-158.

Jennifer L. Hunt, MD; Ronald Fairman, MD; Marc E. Mitchell, MD; Jeffrey P. Carpenter, MD; Michael Golden, MD; Tigran Khalapyan, MD; Megan Wolfe, BS; David Neschis, MD; Ross Milner, MD; Benjamin Scott, BS; Anita Cusack, MSN; Emile R. Mohler, III, MD.

KE Watson, Abrolat ML, Malone LL, Hoeg JM, Doherty T, Detrano R, Demer LL.
Active serum vitamin D levels are inversely correlated with coronary calcification Department of Medicine, Los Angeles School of Medicine, Harbor UCLA

Mauriello A, Sangiorgi G, Palmieri G, Virmani R, Holmes DR, Schwartz RS, Pistolese R, Ippoliti A, Spagnoli LG.
Hyperfibrinogenemia associated with specific histocytological composition and complications of atherosclerotic carotid plaques in patients affected by transient ischemic attacks. Circulation 2000 Feb 22;101(7):744-50

Binder BR, Geiger M.
Clin. Exp. Physiol., University Vienna, Austria
Possible Links between Risk Factors for Cardiovascular Disease: Fibrinogen, Endothelial Cells, Coagulation, and Fibrinolysis

Born GVR.
Fibrinogen in Occlusive Arterial Disease

Smith FB, Lee AJ, Hau CM, Rumley A, Lowe GD, Fowkes FG.
Department of Public Health Sciences, University of Edinburgh, UK.
Plasma fibrinogen, haemostatic factors and prediction of peripheral arterial disease in the Edinburgh Artery Study.
Blood Coagul Fibrinolysis 2000 Jan;11(1):43-50.

Humphries SE, Cook M, Dubowitz M, Stirling Y, Meade TW.
Role of genetic variation at the fibrinogen locus in determination of plasma fibrinogen concentrations.

Bielak LF, Klee GG, Sheedy PF, Turner ST, Schwartz RS, Peyser PA.
Department of Epidermiology, University of Michigan, Ann Arbor 48109, USA.
Association of Fibrinogen with quantity of coronary artery calcification measured by electron beam computed tomography.
Arterioscler Thromb Vasc Biol 2000 Sep;20(9):2167-71..

Sweetnam PM, Thomas HF, Yarnell JW, Beswick AD, Baker IA, Elwood PC.
Fibrinogen, viscosity and the 10-year incidence of ischaemic heart disease. Eur Heart J. 1996 Dec;17(12):1814-20.

Ferrie JE, Shipley MJ, Davey Smith G, Stansfeld SA, Marmot MG.
Fibrinogen, viscosity and the 10 year incidence of ischaemic heart disease. Eur Heart J. 1996 Dec;17(12):1814-20.
Ageno W, Finazzi S, Steidl L, Biotti MG, Mera V, Melzi D'Eril G, Venco A.
Psychological distress as a risk factor for coronary heart disease in the Whitehall II Study. Int J Epidemiol. 2002 Feb;31(1):248-55.
Fowkes FG.
Recent progress in the clinical aspects of fibrinogen. Eur Heart J. 1995 Mar;16 Suppl A:54-91296.
Fibrinogen
Ernst E, et al. Eur Heart J. 1995;16(suppl A):47-53.
Branchi A, et al. Thromb Haemost. 1993;70:241-243
Levenson, J, et al. Arteriosclerosis Thromb Vasc Biol 1995;15:1263-1268.
JW Miller.
Homocysteine and Alzheimer's disease. Nutrition reviews-washington

## HOMOCYSTEINE

Malinow MR
Hyperhomocysteinemia. A common & Esily reversible Rffor atherosclerosis. Circulation 1990;81:2004-2006.
Malinow MR, et al.
Carotid artery intimal-medial wall thickening and plasma homocysteine in asymptomatic adults. Circulation 1993;87:1107-1113.
Malinow MR, et al.
Prevalence of hyperhomocyst(e)inemia in patients with peripheral arterial occlusive disease. Circulation 1989;79:1180-1188
Fallon UB, Elwood P, Ben-Shlomo Y, Ubbink JB, Greenwood R,k Smith GD
Homocysteine and ischaemic stroke in men: the Caerphilly study. Department of Social Medicine, University of Bristol, Bristol, Canynge Hall, Whiteladies Road,k Bristol BS8 2PR, UK.
Young, IS, McAuley DF, Hanratty CG, Johnston GD, McGrath LT.
The effects of oral methionine and homocysteine on endothelial functionf. Heart (british cardiac society).
Rene M. Malinow, Irginia J. Howard, Lloyd E. Chambless, L. Creed Pettigrew, Meir Stampfer, James F. Toole, J. David Spence.
Vitamin intervention for stroke prevention (VISP) trial; Rationale and design. Neuroepidemiology.
Alvarez Sab'in J, Tur'onJ, Montaner J, Malinow R, Codina A
[Plasma Homocysteine levels in patients with transient ischemic attacks] Unidad Cerebrovascular, Hospital General Universitario Vall d'Hebron, Barcelc, Med Clin (Barc), 113(14):531-2 1999 Oct 30.
Verhoef P, Hennekens CH, Malinow MR, Kok FJ, Willett WC, Stampfer M.
A prospective study of plasma homocyst(e)ine and risk of ischemic stroke. Department of Epidemiology and Public Health, Agricultural University, Wageningen, Netherlands. Stoke, 25(10):1924-30 1994 Oct.
Malinow MR.
Hyperhomocyst(e)inemia. A common and easily reversible risk factor for occlusive atherosclerosis. Circulation 81, 2004-2006, 1990.
Malinow MR, Duell PB, Hess DL, Anderson PH, Kruger WD, Phillipson BE, Gluckman RA, Block PC, Upson BM.
Reduction of plasma homocyst(e)ine levels by breakfast cereal fortified with folic acid in patients with coronary heart disease. N Engl J Med 338, 1009-1015, 1998.

_Malinow MR, Bostom AG, Krauss RM._
_Homocyst(e)ine, Diet, and Cardiovascular Diseases._ American Heart Assn. Science Advisory. A Statement for Healthcare Professionals from the Nutrition Committee, American Heart Association. Circulation 99, 178-182, 1999.
_Mehrabi MR, Huber K, Serbecic N, Wild T, Wojta J, Tamaddon F, Morgan A, Ullrich R,k Dietmar Glogar H.U_
Plasma homocysteine in subjects with familial combined hyperlipidemia. Atherosclerosis. 2003 Jan;166(1):111-7.
_Gazzaruso C, Garzaniti A, Giordanetti S, Falcone C, Fratino P._
Elevated homocysteine serum level is associated with low enrichment of homocysteine in coronary arteries of patients with coronary artery disease. Thromb Res. 2002 Sep 1;107(5):189-196.
_Noverhoef P, Pasman WJ, Van Vliet T, Urgert R, Katan MB._
Enhanced risk of thrombotic disease in patients with acquired vitamin B(12) and/or folate deficiency: role of hyperhomocysteinemia Ann Hermatol. 2002.
_Evans M, Roberts A, Rees A._
Homocysteine, folate deprivation and Alzheimer neuropathology. J Alzheimers Dis. 2002 Aug;4(4):261-7.
_Cingozbay BY, Yiginer O, Cebeci BS, Kardesoglu E, Demiralp E, Dincturk M._
Elevated plasma total homocysteine increased the risk of dementia in the elderly. Evid Based Ment Health. 2002 Nov;5(4):126.
_De Bree A, Verschuren WM, Kromhout D, Kluijtmans LA, Blom HJ._
Role of homocysteine for thromboembolic complication in patients with non-valvular atrial fibrillation. Blood Coagul Fibrinolysis. 2002 Oct;13(7): 609-13.
_Tofler GH, D'Agostino RB, Jacques PF, Bostom AG, Lipinska I, Mittleman MA, Selhub J._
Homocysteine determinants and the evidence to what extent homocysteine determines the risk of coronary heart disease. Pharmacol Rev. 2002 Dec;54(4):599-61.
_Burke AP, Fonseca V, Kolodgie F, Zieske A, Fink L, Virmani R._
Association between increased homocysteine levels and impaired fibrinolytic potential: potential mechanism for cardiovascular risk. Thromb Haemost. 2002 Nov;88(5):799-804.
_Eikelboom JW, Hankey GJ, Anand SS, Lofthouse E, Staples N, Baker RI._
Intermediate and severe hyperhomocysteinemia with thrombosis: a study of genetic determinants. Thromb Haemost. 2000 Apr;83(4):554-8.
_Malinow MR, Nieto FJ, Kruger WD, Duell PB, Hess DL, Gluckman RA, Block PC, Holzgang CR, Anderson PH, Seltzer D, Upson B, Lin QR._
The case for mild hyperhomocysteinaemia as a risk factor.
_Konecky N, Malinow MR, Tunick PA, Freedberg RS, Rosenzqeig BP, Katz ES, Hess DL, Upson B, Leung B, Perez J, Kronzon I._
The effects of folic acid supplementation on plasma total homocysteine are modulated by ultivitamin use and methylenetetrahydrofolate reductase genotrypes. Arterioscler Thromb Vasc Biol. 1997 Jun;17(6):1157-62.
_Pellicano R, Oliaro E, Gandolfo N, Aruta E, Mangiardi L, Orzan F, Bergerone S, Rizzetto M, Ponzetto A._
Importance of hyperhomocysteinemia as a risk factor for venous thromboembolism in a Taiwanese population. A case-control study. Thromb Res. 2001 Jun1;102(5):387-95.
_Sierksma A, Van der Gaag MS, Kluft C, Hendriks HF._
Hyperhomocysteinemia and endothelial function in young subjects: effects of vitamin supplementation. Clin Cardiol. 2002 Nov;25(11):495-501.

## STROKE

_Megan C Leary et al._
Incidence of Silent Stroke in the United States. Abstracts International Stroke Conference 2000 32:363-b.

Boers GH.
Association between high homocyst(e)ine and ischemic stroke due to large-and small-artery disease but not of ischemic stroke. Stroke: 2000 May;31(5):1069-75.
Kelly PJ, et al.
Mild-to-moderate hyperhomocyst(e)inemia and risk of stroke. Abstracts of the International Stroke Conference 2000 32:366.
Sillesen H, Neilsen T.
Clinical significance of intraplaque hemorrhage in carotid artery disease. J Neuroimaging, 1998;8:15-19.
Chyi-Huey Bai, et al.
Relations between coagulation profiles, lipid profiles, and factors with risk of first-ever ischemic stroke: a novel case-control study. Abstracts of the International Stroke Conference 2000 32:267-b Poster Presentation. P 156.
Fichtlscherer S, et al.
Elevated C-reactive protein levels and impaired endoth vasoreactivity in patients with coronary artery disease. Circulation (Online) 2000.
Fallon UB, Elwood P, Ben-Shlomo Y, Ubbink JB, Greenwood R,k Smith GD
Homocysteine and ischaemic stroke in men: the Caerphilly study. Department of Social Medicine, University of Bristol, Bristol, Canynge Hall, Whiteladies Road,k Bristol BS8 2PR, UK.
Qizilbash N.
Fibrinogen and cerebrovascular disease. Departmentr of Clinical Geratoloty, University of Oxford
Kalayoglu MV, Libby P, Byrne GI.
Chlamydia pneumoniae in Carotid Artery Atherosclerosis: A Comparison of Its Presence in Atherosclerotic Plaque, Healthy Vessels, and Circulating Leukocytes From the Same Individuals Stroke. 2002 Dec;33(12):2756-61.

**DENTAL, (PERIDONTAL DISEASE)**
Kumari M, Marmot M, Brunner E.
Coronary artery disease and periodontal disease: is there a link? Angiology. 2002 Mar-Apr;53(2):141-8.
Westrich GH, Weksler BB, Glueck CJ, Blumenthal BF, Salvati EA.
Effect of treating periodontitis on C-reactive protein levels: a pilot study. BMC Infect Dis. 2002 Dec 10;2(1):30.
Strachan DPO, Mendall MA, Carrington D, Butland BK, Yarnell JW, Sweetnam PM, Elwood PC.
Effect of treating periodontitis on C-reactive protein levels: a pilot study. BMC Infect Dis. 2002 Dec 10;2(1):30. Secondary prevention by raising HDL cholesterol and reducing triglycerides in patients with coronary artery disease: the Bezafibrate. Infarction Prevention (BIP) study.

**CYTOMEGALOVIRUS, CMV**
Kendall TJ, Wilson JE, Radio SJ, Kandolf R, Gulizia JM, Winters GL Costanzo-Nordin MR, Malcom GT, Thieszen SL, Miller LW, et al
Cytomegalovirus associated inflammatory heart muscle disease. Scand J Infect Dis Suppl. 1993;88:135-48.
Wink K. Schmitz H.
Cytomegalovirus and other herpesviruses: do they have a role in the development of accelerated coronary arterial disease in human heart allografts? J Heart Lung Transplant. 1992 May-Jun;11(3 Pt 2):S14-20.
Smieja M, Cronin L, Levine M, Goldsmith CH, Yusuf S, Mahony JB.
Cytomegalovirus myocarditis. Am Heart J. 1980 Nov;100(5):667-72.
Veerkamp MJ, de Graaf J, den Heijer M, Blom HJ, Stalenhoef AF.
Chlamydia pneumoniae, herpes simplex virus type 1.

## HELICOBACTER PYLORI

The association of seropositivity to Helicobacter pylori, Chlamydia pneumoniae, and cytomegalovirus with risk of cardiovascular disease: a prospective study. J Am Coll Cardiol. 2002 Oct 16:40(8):1408-13.

Maisch B, schonian U, Crombach M, Wendl I, Bethge C, Herzum M, Klein HH.
Chronic infections and atherosclerosis. J Med Assoc Thai. 2001 Dec;84 Suppl 3:S650-7.203.

Patel P, Mendall MA, Carrington D, et al.
Association of Helicobacter pylori and Chlamydia pneumoniae infections with coronary heart disease and cardiovascular risk factors. Brit Med J 1995, 311:711-714.

Cushman M, Lemaitre RN, Kuller LH, Psaty BM, Macy EM, Sharrett AR, Tracy RP.
Treatment of Helicobacter pylori and Chlamydia pneumoniae infections decreases fibrinogen plasma level in patients with ischemic heart disease. Circulation. 1999 Mar 30;99(12):1555-9. Cushman M, Lemaitre RN, Kuller LH, Psaty BM, Macy EM, Sharrett AR, Tracy RP.

Hopkins PN, Stephenson S, Wu LL, Riley WA, Xin Y, Hunt SC.
Ischemic cardiovascular disease and Helicobacter pylori. Where is the link? J Cardiovasc Surg (Torino), 2000 Dec;41(6):829-33.

## DVT

Kannelk WB, Wolf PA, Castelli WP, D'Agostino RB,
Deep vein thrombosis and its prevention in patients with acute myocardial infarction. Cor Vasa. 1988;30(5):345-51.

Kleishadi R, Zadegan NS, Naderi GA, Asgary S, Bashardoust N.
Prevalence and clinical correlates of peripheral arterial disease in the Framingham Offspring Study. Am Heart J. 2002 Jun;143(6):961-5

## AlZHEIMERS

Rosenberg IH, Selhub J, Jacques PF, Morris MS.
Hyperhomocysteinemia associated with poor recall in the third National Health and Nutrition Examination Survey.
American journal of clinical nutrition

Gottfries CG, Regland B.
Earlyl diagnosis of cognitive impairment in the elderly with the focus on Alzheimer's disease.
Journal of neural transmission.

## STRESS

Whitty CJ, Brunner EJ, Shipley MJ, Hemingway H, Marmot MG.
Differences in biological risk factors for cardiovascular disease between three ethnic groups in the Whitehall II study. Atherosclerosis 1999 Feb;142(2):279-86. International Centre for Health and Society, Department of Epidermiolgy and Public Health, University College London, UK.

Stansfeld SA, Fuhrer R, Shupley MJ, Marmot MG.
Department of Psychiatry, Barts and the London, Queen Mary's School of Medicine and Dentistry.
Health effects of anticipation of job change and non-employment: longitudinal data from the Whitehall II Study. BMJ (England), Nov 11 1995, 311(7015) p1264-9.

Whitty CJ, Brunner EJ, Shipley MJ, et al.
Differences in biological risk factors for cardiovascular disease between three ethnic groups in the Whitehall II study. Atherosclerosis (Irland), Feb 1999, 142(2) p279-86.

Fuhrer R, Head J, Marmot MG.
Social position, age, and memory performance in the Whitehall II Study. Ann N Y Acad Sci (United States), 1999, 896 p359-62.

Stansfeld SA, Fuhrer R, Shipley MJ, et al
Psychological distress as a risk factor for coronary; heart disease in the Whitehall II Study. Int J Epidemiol (England), Feb 2002, 31(1) p248-55.

Brunner EJ, Marmot MG, Nanchahal K, et al.
Social inequality in coronary risk: central obesity and the metabolic syndrome. Evidence from the Whitehall II study. Diabetologia (Germany), Nov 1997, 40(11) p1341-9.
Hemingway H, Nicholson A, Stafford M, Roberts R, Marmot M.
Department of Epidemiology and Public Health, University College London Medical School, England.
The impact of socioeconomic status on health functioning as assessed by the SF-36 questionnaire: the Whitehall II Study.
Am J Public Health 1997 Sep;87(9):1484-90.

**REGRESSION OF HEART DISEASE**
Superko HR, Krauss RM.
Coronary artery disease regression. Convincing evidence for the benefit of aggressive lipoprotein management. Circulation 90: 1056-1069. Lawrence Berkeley Laboratory, Life Science Division, University of California, Berkeley.
Stary HC.
The development of calcium deposits in atherosclerotic lesions and their persistence after lipid regression. Am J Cardiol. 2001;88:16E-19E.
Strong JP, Bhattacharyya AK, Eggen DA, et al.
Long-term induction and regression of diet-induced atherosclerotic lesions in rhesus monkeys, I:morphological and chemical evidence for regression of lesions in the aorta and carotid and peripheral arteries. Arterioscler Thromb. 1994;958-965.
The Potential for Regression and Applications in the Cardiac Rehabilitation Setting. In Clinical Cardiac Rehibilation: A Cardiologist's Guide ed. FJ Pashkow and WA Dafor, Williams & Wilkins, 1998; pp.327-364.
Superko HR.
Atherosclerosis Regression Trials: An Overview. Lipids & Atherogenesis 1991;1(3):1-4.
Superko HR.
Banerjee AK, Pearson J, Gilliland EL, Goss D, Lewis JD, Stirling Y, Meade TW.
A six year prospective study of fibrinogen and other risk factors associated with mortality in stable claudicants.
Thromb Haemost 1992 Sep 7;68(3):261-3.

**DIABETES MELLITUS**
Zachary T. Bloomgarden, MD.
Insulin Resistance: Does Treatment decrease Cardiovascular Disease Risk?
Li H, Lewis A, Brodsky S, Rieger R, Iden C, Golingorsky MS.
Homocysteine induces 3-hydroxy-3-methlglutaryl coenzyme a reductable vascular endothelial cells: a mechanism for development of atherosclerosis. Circulation, 105(9): 1037-43 2002.
Bruno G, Cavallo-Perin P, Bargero G, Borra M, E'Erfrico N, Macchia G, Pagano G.
Department of Internal Medicine, University of Turin, Turin, Italy
Hyperfibrinogenemia and metabolic syndrome in type 2 diabetes: a population-based study. Diabes Metab Res Rev 2001 Mar-Apr;17(2):124-30
Berthezene F.
Aruna D, Pradhan, MD, MPH, JoAnn E. Manson, MD, DrPH, Nader Rifai, PhD, Julie E. Buring, ScD, Paul M. Ridker, MD, MPH.
C-Reactive Protein, Interleukin 6, and Risk of Developing Type 2 Diabetes Mellitus.
The management of diabetic dyslipidemia. Program and abstracts of the 37th Annual Meeting of the European Association for the Study of Diabetes (EASD); September 9-13, 2001; Glasgow, United Kingdom. Symposium.
Diabetes Atherosclerosis Intervention Study Group. Effect of fenofibrate on progression of coronary-artery disease in type 2 diabetes: the Diabetes Atherosclerosis Intervention Study, a randomized study. Lancet. 2001;357:905-910.

*McCarty MF*
*Interluken-6 as a central mediator of cardiovascular risk associated with chronic inflammation, smoking, diabetes, and visceral obesity, down-regulation with essential fatty acids, ethanol and pentoxifylline. Med Hypotheses 1999 May;52(5):465-77.*

## LIPOPROTEIN SUBFRACTIONS
*Superko HR.*
*Inclusion of lipoprotein subfactions among efficacy parameters. AM J Cardiology. 1998; 14:20-23.*

*Superko HR.*
*Small Dense LDL. The new coronary artery disease risk factor and how it is changing the treatment of CAD. Preventive Cardiology 1998; 16-24.*

*Superko HR.*
*Did Grandma give you heart disease? The new battle against coronary artery disease. AM J Cardiology 1998;82-34Q-64Q.*

*Superko HR, Dunn HP.*
*Sophisticated Metabolic Atherosclerosis Diagnosis and Treatment for Coronary Artery Disease:*
*New Aspects of Cardiovascular Risk Factors Including Small, Dense LDL, Homocysteinemia, and Lp (a). Current Opinions in Cardiology 1995;10:347-354.*

*Superko HR, Greenland P, Manchester RA, Andreadis NA, Schectman G, Hendriksen West N, Haskell WH.*
*Effectiveness of low dose copestipol therapy in patients with moderate ghpercholesterolemia. Am J Cardiology 1992; 70:135-140.*

*Arefieva TL, Krasnikova TL.*
*Institute of Experimental Cardiology, Cardiology Research Center, Moscow, Russia. Monocytic cell adhesion to intact and plasmin-modified fibrinogen: possible involvement of Mac-1 (CD11b/CD18) and ICAM-1 (CD54). J Cell Physiol 2001 Sep;188(3):403-9.*

*Ridker, PM, Rifai N, Rose L, Buring JE, Cook NR.*
*Inflammatory bio-markers and cardiovascular risk prediction. J Intern Med. 2002 Oct;252(4):283-94.*

*Koenig W.*
*Comparison of C-reactive protein and low-density lipoprotein cholesterol levels in the prediction of first cardiovascular events. N Engl J Med. 2002 Nov 14;347(20):1557-65.*

*Whincup PH, Danesh J, Walker M, Lennon L, Thomson A, Appleby P, Rumley A, Lowe GD.*
*Insulin resistance, heart disease and inflammation. Identifying the 'at-risk' patient: the earlier the better? The role of inflammatory markers. Int J Clin Pract Suppl. 2002 Oct;(132):23-30.*

*Ann Neurol.*
*Inflammatory Marker Linked to Long-Term Risk of Dementia 2002;52:168-174.*

*Eva Lindmark, Mmed, Erik Diderholm, MD, Lars Wallentin, MD, Phd, Ageneta Siegbahn, MD, PhD.*
*Relationship Between Interleukin 6 and Mortality in Patients With Unstable Coronary Artery Disease.*

*Kannel WB.*
*Hazards, risks and threats of heart disease form the early stages to symptomatic coronary heart disease and cardiac failure. Cardiovasc Drugs Ther 1997;11 Suppl:199-212[review].*

*Gotto AM Jr.*
*Triglyceride as a risk factor for coronary artery disease. Am J Cardiol 1998;1998;82:Q22-5 [review].*

Schaefer FJ, Lamon-Fava S, Ordovas JM, et al.
Factors associated with low and elevated plasma high density lipoprotein cholesterol and apolipoprotein A-1 levels in the Framingham Offspring Study. J Lipid Res 1994;35:871.
Hu FB, Stampfer MJ, Rimm E, et al.
Dietary fat and coronary heart disease: a comparison of approaches for adjusting for total energy intake and modeling repeated dietary measurements. Am J Epidemiol 1999;149:531
Kinosian B, Glick H, Garland G.
Cholesterol and coronary heart disease: predicting risks by levels and ratios. Ann Intern Med 1994;121:641-7,
Kannel WB.
Hazards, risks, and threats of heart disease from the early stages to symptomatic coronary heart disease and cardiac failure. Cardiovasc Drugs Ther 1997;11 Suppl:199-212
Undas A, Brummel KE, Musial J, Mann KG, Szczeklik A.
Omega-3 Fatty Acids & Bipolar Disorder
Highlights of a Lecture by Andrew L. Stoll, M.D., Director, Psychopharmacology Research Laboratory, McLean Hospital June 9, 1999.
Whimcup PH, Refsum H, Perry IJ, Morris R, Walker M, Lennon L, Thomso Ueland PM, Ebrahim SB
Serum total homocysteine and coronary heart disease: prospective study in middle aged men. Heart, 82(4):448-54 1999 Oct.

## CLOTTING,

Steve E. Humphries, PhD.
Epidemiology of Arterial Thrombotic Disease
British Heart Foundation Professor Cardiovascular Genetics
Atherosclerosis
Herbert C. Stary, MD, Chari, A. Bleakley Chandler, MD, Robert E. Dinsmore, MD, Valentin Fuster, MD, PhD, Seymour Glagov, MD, William Insull, Jr, MD, Michael E. Rosefeld, PhD, Colin J. Schwartz, MD, Williams D. Wagner, PhD, Robert W. Wissler, PhD, MD.
Hypercoagulability: Clinical Assessment and Treatment from Southern Medical Journal.
A Definition of Advanced Types of Atherosclerotic Lesions and a Histological Classification of Atherosclerosis
Doevendans PA, Jukema W, Spiering W, Defesche JC, Kastelein JJ.
Molecular genetics and gene expression in atherosclerosis. Int J Cardiol, 80(2-3):L 161-72 2001.
Riodan Schilling V, Marin Ortuno F, Pineda Rocamora J, Climent Paya VE, Martinez JG, Marco Vera P, de Teresa Parreno L, Sogorb Garri F.
Serviceo de Cardiologia, Hospital General Universitario de Alicante. Thrombogenic and endothelial damage markers in patients with ischemic systolic impairment. Rev Esp Cardiol 2001 Oct;54(10):1155-60.
Blankenberg S, Tiret L, Bickel C, Peetz D, Cambien F, Meyer J, Rupprecht HF.
Fibrinogen, Viscosity and the 10 year incidence of ischaemic heart disease.
Hemostatic factors as predictors of coronary events and total mortality: The FINRISK '92 Hemostasis Study
Arterioscler Thromb Vasc Biol (United States), Feb 1 2002, 22(2)p353-8.
Douglas E. Vaughan, MD.
Angiotensin II, Fibrinolysis, and Vascular Homeostasis.
Lowe GD, Fowkes FG, Dawes J, Donnan PT, Lennie SE, Housley E.
Blood viscosity, fibrinogen, and activation of coagulation and leukocytes in peripheral arterial disease and the normal population in the Edinburgh Artery Study.
Circulation. 1993 Jun;87(6):1915-20.

Neil Bramson, MD, Simeon Abramson, MD, Department of Education and Research, Baptist Regional Cancer Institute, Baptist Medical Center, Jacksonville, Fla.
Hypercoagulability: Clinical Assessment and Treatment From Southerrn Medical Journal.
Simvastatin depresses blood clotting by inhibiting activation of prothrombi V, and factor XIII and by enhancing factor Va inactivation. Circulation, 103(18): 2248-53.
Szczeklik A, Undas A, Musial J, Gajewski P, swadzba J, Jankowski M.
Antithrombotic actions of statins. Med Sci Monit, 7(6): 1381-5 0.
Salomaa V, Rasi V, Kulathinal S, Vahtera E, Jauhiainen M, Ehnholm C, Pekkanen J.
Department of Epidemiology and Health Promotion, KTL-National Public Health Institute, Helsinki. Hemostatic factors as predictors of coronary events and total mortality: The FINRISK '92 Hemostasis Study.

## LP (a)
Superko HR, Krauss RM.
Coronary Artery Disease Regression. Convincing Evidence for the Benefit of Aggressive Lipoprotein Management. Circulation 1994;90:1057-1069.
Superko HR.
New Aspects of Cardiovascular Risk Factors Including Small, Dense LDL, Homocysteinemia, and Lp)a). Current Opinons in Cardiology 1995;10:347-354.
Gaubatz JW, et al.
Polymorphic forms of human apolipoprotein(a): inheritance and relationship of their molecular weights to plasma levels of lipoprotein(a). J Lipid Research 1'990;31:603-613.

## TROPONINS
Braunwald E, et al.
ACC/AHA guidelines for the management of patients with unstable angina and non-ST-segment elevation myocardial infarction. A report of the American College of Cardiology/ American Heart Association Task Force on Practice Guidelines (Committee on the Management of Patients With Unstable Angina). J Am Coll Cardiol 2000;36:970
Nomenclature and criteria for diagnosis of ischemic heart disease. Report of the Joint International Society and Federation of Cardiology/World Health Organization task force on standardization of clinical nomenclature. Circulation 1979;59:607.
Ohman EM, et al.
Cardiac troponin T levels for risk stratification in acute myocardial ischemia. GUSTOIIA Investigators. N Engl J Med 1996;335:1333.
Hamm, CW, et al.
Emergency room triage of patients with acute chest pain by means of rapid testing for cardiac troponin T or troponin I. N Engl J Med 1997;337:1648.
Keffer JH.
Myocardial markers of injury. Evolution and insights [review]. Am J Clin Patho/ 1996;105:305.
Myocardial infarction redefined—a consensus document of The Joint European Society of Cardiology/American College of Cardiology Committee for the redefinition of myocardial infarction. J Am Coll Cardiol 2000;36:959.

## AORTIC VALVE
Medscape Cardiology. Cardiovascular Disease, Aortic Valve Sclerosis, [Medscape Cardiology, 1999.
Juvonen J, Juvonen T, Laurila A, et al.
Can degenerative aortic valve stenosis be related by persistent Chlamydia pneumoniae infection? Ann Intern Med 1998, 128:741-744.

## D-Dimer of Fibrin
Lee AJ, Fowkes FG, Lowe GD, Rumley AU.
Fibrin D-dimer, haemostatic factors and peripheral arterial disease.

*Thromb Haemost. 1995 Sep;75(3)828-32*
*Lowe GD, Yarnell JW, Rumley A, et al.*
C-reactive protein, fibrin D-dimer, and incident ischemic heart disease in the Speedwell study: are inflammation and fibrin turnover linked in patheogenesis?
*Arterioscler Thromb Vasc Biol (United States), Apr 2001,21(4)p603-10.*
*Lowe, GD, Yarnell JW, Rumley A, et al.*
C-reactive protein, fibrin D-dimer, and incident ischemic heart disease in the Speedwell study: are inflammation and fibrin turnover linked in pathogenesis?
*Arterioscler Thromb Vasc Biol, (United States), Apr 2001, 21(4)p603-10*
*Mills JD, Mansfield MW, Grant PJ*
Tissue plasminogen activator, fibrin D-dimer, and insulin resistance in the relatives of patients with premature coronary artery disease.
*Arterioscler Thromb Vasc Biol (United States), Apr 1 2002, 22(4) p704-9*
*Koenig W..*
Hemostatic factors and the risk of myocardial infraction or sudden death in patients with angina pectoris, European Concerted Action on Thrombosis and Disabilities Angina Pectoris Study Group. N Engl J Med. 1995 Mar 9;332(10):635-41.
*Juhan-Vague I, Renucci JF, Grimaux M, et al.*
Thrombin-activatable fibrinolysis inhibitor antigen levels and cardiovascular risk factors.
*Arterioscler Thromb Vasc Biol (United States), Sep 2000, 20(9) p2156-61.*
*Libby P, Sinon DI.*
Inflammation and thrombosis: the clot thickens. Circulation, 2001;103:1718-1720.

## SLEEP APNEA

*Blake GJ, Ridker PM.*
Independent contribution of psychological factors to fibrin turnover in subjects with sleep apnoea and/or systemic hypertension. Clin Sci (Lond). 2002 Oct;103(4):331-7.
*Javahari, Liming*
Sleep Apnea in 81 ambulatory Male Patients with Stable Heart Failure, Circulation 1998
Women snorers, diabetes and insulin resistance
*American Journal of Epidimiology, 2002*
*American Academy of Pediactrics, 4/2000.*

## SUPPLEMENTS, L-Carnitine, Fish oil, Coenzyme Q10, Taurine, Green tea,

*Rahman K, et al.*
Dietary Supplementation with Aged Garlic Extract Inhibits ADP-Induced Platelet Aggregation in Humans. J Nutr 2000 Nov;130(11):2662-2665.
*Kang WS, et al.*
Antithrombotic activities of green tea catechins and (-)-epigallocatechin gallate. Throm Res 1999 Nov 1;96(3):229-37.
*Vyshevskii Ash, et al.*
[The role of platelets in the protective effect of a combination of vitamins A, E, C and P in thrombinemia]. Gematol Transfuziol 1995 Sep-Oct;40(5):9-11.
*Flaten H, et al.*
Fish-oil concentrate: effects on variables related to cardiovascular disease. Am J Clin Nutr 1990 Aug;52(2):300-6.
*Baggio E, Gandini R, Plancher AC, Passeri M, Carmosino G.*
Italian multicenter study on the safety and efficacy of coenzyme Q10 as adjunct therapy in heart failure. COQ10 Drug Suveillance Investigators. Mol Aspects Med, 15 Suppl(-HD-:s287-94 1994.
*Kritchevsky SB.*
Bete-carotene, carotenoids and the prevention of coronary heart disease. J Nutr 1999;129:5-8 [review].

_Palace VP, Khaper N, Qin Q, Singal PK._
_Antioxidant potentials of vitamin A and carotenoids and their relevance to heart disease._
_Free Radic Biol Med 1999;26:746-61_
_Bonow RO, Carabello B, de Leon AC Jr, et al._
_ACC/AHA guidelines for the management of patients with valvular heart disease: a report_
_of the American College of Cardiology/American Heart Association Task Force on Practice_
_Guidelines (Committee on Management of Patients With Valvular Heart Disease). J AM_
_Coll Cardiol. 1998;32:1486-588._
_Hofman-Bang C, Rehnqvist N, Swedberg K, Wiklund I, Astr om H._
_Coenzyme Q10 as an adjunctive in the treatment of chronic congestive heart failure. The_
_Q10 Study Group. J Card Fail, 1(2):101-7 1995 Mar._
_Pion PD, Sanderson SL, Kittelson MD._
_The effectiveness of taurine and l-carnitine in dogs with heart disease._
_Vet Clin North Am Small Anim Pract, 28(6):1495-514, ix 1998 Nov._
_Freeman LM._
_Interventional nutrition for cardiac disease. Clin Tech Small Anim Pract, 13(4):232-7 1998_
_Nittynen L, Nurminen ML, Korpela R, Vapaatalo H._
_Role of arginine, taurine and homocysteine in cardiovascular diseases. Valio Ltd, Research_
_and Development, Helsinki, finland. Ann Med, 31(5):318-26 1999 Oct._
_Sanbe A, Tanonaka K, Niwano Y, Takeo S._
_Improvement of cardiac function and nyocardial energy metabolism of rats with chronic_
_heart failure by long-term coenzyme Q10 treatment._
_Sayed-Ahmed MM, Shouman SA, Rezk BM, Khalifa MH, Osman AM, El-Merzabani_
_Propionyl-L-carnitine as potential protective agent against adriamycin-induced impairement_
_of fatty acid beta-oxidation in isolated heart mitochondria. Pharmacol Res, 41(2):143-50_
_2000 Feb._
_Sethi R, Dhalla KS, Ganguly PK, Ferrari R, Dhalla NS._
_Beneficial effects of propionyl L-carnitine on sarcolemmal changes in congestive heart failure_
_due to myocardial infarction. Cardiovasc Res, 42(3):607-15 1999 Jun._
_Rizos I._
_Three-year survival of patients with heart failure caused by dilated cardiomyopathy and L-_
_carnitine administration. University of Athens Medical School, Greece. Am Heart J 139(2_
_Pt 3):S120-3 2000 Feb._
_Kikuo Arakawa, MD, Hans R. Brunner, MD, Bryan Williams, MD, Douglas E. Vaughan,_
_MD, W. Robert Taylor, MD, PhD, Hiroyuki Koike, PhD, Joel M. Neutel, MD, Michael A._
_Weber, MD._
_Pressure, Platelets, and Plaque: The Central Role of Angiotensin II in Cardiovascular_
_Pathology._
_McCarty MF._
_Fish oil and other nutritional adjuvants for treatment of congestive heart failure. Med_
_Hypotheses, 46(4):400-6 1996 Apr._
_Broderick TL, Quinney HA, Lopaschuk GD._
_L-carnitine increases glucose metabolism and mechanical function following ischaemia in_
_diabetic rat heart._
_Paradies G, Petrosillo G, Gadaleta MN, Ruggiero FM._
_The effect of aging and acetyl-L-carnitine on the pyruvate transport and oxidation in rat_
_heart mitochondria._

_Sources: Medline, Cardiosource, Medscape, Introvieve, medical journals including Lancet,_
_Journals of the American Heart Association._